Nurturing Maternity Staff is a powerfully empathic account of how it feels to work in maternity with chronic work overload, staff shortages and increasing complexity of birthing challenges. It is a book which embodies the compassion it advocates in its pages, written by someone who has had the courage to speak up for the many maternity staff who feel afraid or abandoned in workplaces that have too often lost their connection with the core healthcare value of compassion.

Professor Michael West CBE, Senior Visiting Fellow, The King's Fund, Professor of Organizational Psychology, Lancaster University, Emeritus Professor, Aston University

Nurturing Maternity Staff by Dr Jan Smith is clearly informed by years of experience supporting families afflicted by birth related-trauma and maternity staff overwhelmed with work related stress, anxiety or perceived guilt. At the same time as being highly informative, Jan's compassion and her storytelling abilities using real scenarios has made this an engaging read.

Professor Hora Soltani MBE, Professor in Maternal and Infant Health, Sheffield Hallam University

With mental health consistently being the most cited reason for staff absence throughout the NHS, more must be done to address this. *Nurturing Maternity Staff* outlines how to effectively support the mental health and wellbeing of maternity staff, ensuring they can come to work in a psychologically safe environment and deliver the best care possible.
The strategies in this book will be key in not only improving the experiences of maternity staff, but also providing safer maternity care overall.

Dr Rosena Allin-Khan, MP, Shadow Cabinet Member for Mental Health

Pregnancy, childbirth and the early years is a critical time; the foundation to physical and psychological health and wellbeing when secure attachments and positive relationships are formed. Maternity care workers play a crucial role in enabling these processes yet pressures resulting from inadequate staffing levels, organisational dysfunction, fear and the current pandemic all contribute to staff feeling burnt out, overwhelmed and distressed. Change is urgent if we are to curb the flow of midwives and obstetricians leaving their professions, and the number of women and birthing people experiencing a traumatic birth experience or negative outcomes.

Nurturing Maternity Staff lays out the facts clearly, drawing on research evidence including heart-rendering accounts from individuals highlighting the harm being caused to the lives of health professionals and consequently to those they serve.

It is an urgently needed and accessible resource for all working in direct contact with families, leaders at all levels, CEOs responsible for maternity services and politicians. If we are truly committed to improving safety and health outcomes for mothers and babies then we must tend to the wellbeing of maternity staff – before it's too late.

Sheena Byrom, RM, OBE, Director of All4Maternity

In this brilliant and timely book, Jan Smith shares real-life colleagues' experiences, together with practical tips to help us to be kind to ourselves and to each other. In so doing, she makes a unique and hugely valuable contribution to tackling trauma, stress and burnout in the workplace. Jan Smith's incredible insight into why and how to nurture staff and create a positive culture is a 'must read' for all of us working in maternity services.

Dr Alison Wright, Consultant Obstetrician & Gynaecologist, Royal Free Hospital, National Specialty Advisor for Obstetrics NHS England and NHS Improvement, GMC council member, UK representative FIGO safe motherhood and PPH working group

NURTURING MATERNITY STAFF

How to tackle trauma, stress
and burnout to create a positive
working culture in the NHS

Jan Smith

pinter
&
martin

Nurturing Maternity Staff: How to tackle trauma, stress and burnout to create a positive working culture in the NHS

First published in the UK by Pinter & Martin 2021
reprinted 2022

Copyright © Jan Smith 2021

ISBN 978-1-78066-735-5

Also available as an ebook and audio book

Author photograph by Emma Ledwith

Illustration page 138: Salma Price-Nell at thesalsacreative.com

British Library Cataloguing-in-Publication Data
A catalogue record for this book is available from the British Library

Printed in the EU by Hussar

This book has been printed on paper that is sourced and harvested from sustainable forests and is FSC accredited

Pinter & Martin Ltd
6 Effra Parade
London SW2 1PS

pinterandmartin.com

CONTENTS

AUTHOR'S NOTE

Many of the experiences and content in this book are difficult to read. Please put the book down and reach out to someone for support if you are struggling. This could be a friend, family member, colleague, therapist, or healthcare professional.

This book is not meant to diagnose any symptoms you might be experiencing, or replace any support you are currently receiving. The suggested strategies are to inspire you to create your own, and begin a dialogue with friends, family, colleagues, or your organisation about what might work best to support your mental wellbeing.

Throughout the book the term 'maternity staff' is used to encompass the range of maternity professionals working in this sector. I have also used the term 'women and birthing people' to acknowledge transgender and gender non-conforming people who give birth. The term 'Trust' is used throughout the UK to denote the NHS services and organisations. In the context of this book it is the NHS organisation or service providing maternity input.

Introduction

MATERNITY STAFF MATTER

Over the years, I have been fortunate to witness the passion, commitment, and dedication of many maternity staff in providing compassionate and patient-led care. Often, those who work in maternity services have been nurtured and nourished by their organisation, and they have felt valued and respected by their leaders.

Yet this is not the state of maternity care consistently across the country. Currently, we are haemorrhaging midwives, and the workforce is not only emotionally depleted, but many are also psychologically traumatised, with some feeling they have no alternative but to take their own lives or leave the profession.

Birth rates in England are continuing to fall, but maternity staff are supporting more women requiring complex care. The retention rate of midwives is at a crisis point, with the Royal College of Midwives (RCM)[1] estimating a shortage of 3,500 full-time midwives in England. Although 2,132 midwives graduated from English universities in 2016–17, the midwifery workforce increased by only 67 to 21,601. This means that one newly qualified midwife enters the NHS for every 30 who newly qualify, with attrition rates at their greatest in the first two years post-qualifying.[2] This is a dire situation. While increasing university places on medical and midwifery courses is helpful, it's not the whole solution. I believe we need to pause, reflect and question why this is happening.

Some research has reported that of nearly 2,000 midwives questioned, most were experiencing personal burnout, and over half were burnt out due to work.[3] There were also high levels of stress, anxiety, and depression in over one-third of midwives. Compared to midwives in other countries, the emotional wellbeing of UK midwives is worse.[4] This is particularly the case for midwives under the age of 40, having less than 10 years of experience, working in a clinical midwifery setting, and having a disability. When asked, midwives discussed how a lack of support at work, inappropriate staffing levels, and not providing the quality of care they wanted to all contributed to them feeling this way.[4,5] Midwife means '[to be] with woman', but if midwives are emotionally exhausted and not feeling supported, they will inevitably struggle to provide compassionate and sensitive care, which is crucial to the wellbeing of childbearing women and birthing people.[6]

It can typically take over 10 years to fully qualify as an obstetrician. For most, the journey requires commitment and many personal sacrifices, as evidenced in Adam Kay's bestselling book *This Is Going To Hurt*. He reports the highs and lows of his life in an overstretched NHS as an overwhelmed young doctor. The book ends with him describing a case in which an unforeseen complication with a patient's pregnancy results in a tragic outcome, and consequently he leaves the profession. Some might think this is perhaps an extreme response, but Kay's experience is not unique. As I read his book, I could see that he was suffering from post-traumatic stress, which he openly admitted to after publication.

Obstetrics and gynaecology staff are not exempt from experiencing work-related trauma. Two in three reported experiencing a traumatic work-related event in a study of 728 trainee clinicians.[7] Unsurprisingly, those with higher post-traumatic stress disorder (PTSD) levels had lower levels of job satisfaction and had more experiences of work-related traumatic events. These trauma symptoms were associated with burnout, which meant that clinicians behaved in a more depersonalised way towards women and birthing people. In response to experiencing these trauma symptoms, many trainees reduced their working hours, and over half were considering leaving obstetrics or the medical profession. Similarly, some consultants considered changing speciality, moving away from clinical practice, or leaving the medical profession altogether.

Imagine, after all the sacrifices and commitment required to qualify as an obstetrician, having to consider changing job or leaving the profession! We urgently need to think about how best to support all healthcare staff, irrespective of their position or grade. Whether the clinicians had experienced a work-related trauma or not, most of them discussed the need for specific trauma support and mandatory training to shift the culture from one of blame to one of support.[7]

I have described the emotional wellbeing of maternity staff before the Covid-19 pandemic of 2019 hit. Evidence of the full impact of the pandemic on maternity staff is still accruing and the ramifications will be felt well into the future. Anecdotally, maternity teams have shared with me how they have come together and supported one another, normalising the challenges working in a pandemic has brought. Others have found that when they have been involved in a serious incident during Covid, it has had more of a detrimental impact on their mental wellbeing than it would have beforehand, and many have found it a struggle to cope even if they were previously able to do so. Most staff have found it difficult to accept that the regular care they would normally provide for women and birthing people has been compromised, while also navigating their anxieties about catching and transmitting Covid-19 to their families.

Although many NHS workplaces have wellbeing initiatives designed to reduce burnout and stress, these have little impact on improving the wellbeing of many staff. Some evidence suggests that this is because the interventions are targeted at the individual level rather than at an organisational level.[8] Maternity staff work in a system. If the system stretches and drains an individual to the point where they have little left to give, not only is the emotional wellbeing of that member of staff going to be compromised, but so is the care they can provide to those they are trying to support.

There are, of course, examples of good practice, where staff feel supported and valued in their work. However, the conversation and focus need to change. Staff should *expect* to work in a psychologically safe environment that can 'hold' them when facing work-related challenges, rather than feel lucky if they happen to work in such a team, department, or organisation.

Part of my work involves supporting families impacted by birth-related trauma and maternity staff impacted by work-related trauma. For me, these are two sides of the same coin. Many maternity staff find it impossible to switch off from work, and understandably engage in less helpful behaviours which help them do this, like excessive alcohol and drug use. In the short term this might work, but the long-term consequences are unsustainable. These behaviours could be symptomatic of staff needing and wanting ways to manage the emotional impact of working in a challenging environment.

Years are spent training staff on how to provide woman-centred care to deliver babies safely. But there is a limited focus on learning ways to minimise the impact of working in an emotionally challenging environment. For many, the ideal version of how they thought their role would be might never come to fruition because of a lack of resources, a bullying working environment, or other factors that take staff away from providing the type of care they want to. This has an impact on maternity professionals' physical and mental wellbeing.

Countless times I have sat and listened to staff talk about their anxieties, stress, trauma, moral injuries, worries, and guilt. Their shame at needing help is palpable, with many coming to see me 'in secret', hiding their feelings from colleagues, their employer, family, and friends. Maternity professionals often discuss the impact a toxic culture of bullying has on them. Others share the workload pressures, not feeling valued, and the ripple effect on their health, relationships, and family life.

I have difficult conversations frequently in my work; that is part of what I do. This book is the beginning of another one of these. I hope that it will raise awareness and highlight that working in maternity care can be emotionally demanding. Alongside the extensive skills and knowledge maternity professionals must acquire, they also need to be supported to work in a challenging and ever-changing healthcare system.

Despite the difficulties faced by maternity staff, there are ways to mitigate the impact of them and facilitate a valued and fulfilling career for those who undoubtedly deserve it.

1

MENTAL WELLBEING
IN MATERNITY

'There is no health without mental health.'

The World Health Organization

Everyone has 'off' days when it might feel like a struggle to get going, or they feel low in mood or irritable. For some, a few days of struggling might turn into feelings that are difficult to manage and are pervasive, influencing their thinking and how they behave towards themselves and others. Over time, the way they experience the world alters.

This chapter aims to outline some typical mental health difficulties maternity staff might face and promote the importance of checking in with themselves and others. It encourages staff to seek support (from a professional, a family member, a colleague, or a friend). This is particularly important given the increasing strain placed on some parts of maternity services and the message that 'resilience' is key to the wellbeing of staff.

There is no evidence that I can find that current maternity staff are more or less able to cope with work pressures than those that went before them. However, 'resilience training' seems to be popular at the moment. I appreciate that the intention is to support staff to manage the pressures and workload they face. However, the perception of staff that have attended training, which they have shared with me, ranges from a subtle feeling that they are somehow lacking, to an overt feeling that they're 'not tough enough' to work in maternity services, or they 'aren't cut out for this job'. Whether resilience is seen as a personality trait or the ability to cope with adversity, staff absorb into their psyche that they are not 'enough' in some way.

Many definitions of resilience emphasise that it is not only the ability to survive, but also to adapt. I have learned that resilience is an ability to learn from difficult conditions and integrate this into an individual's learning, but that it also relies on several factors: context, the environment, and the individual. By way of example, Sam, a consultant obstetrician, shares her experience:

> 'I love what I do, I really do. To many of my colleagues, I think they would probably describe me as a very resilient person if they had to. I'm able to work through a busy clinic, support women who are distressed quite competently and manage some pretty complex obstetric cases. However, I recently moved to a different hospital. I didn't know how the appointment system worked, I couldn't log on to my emails, and my clinic overran by two hours. I sat in the toilets, trying to calm myself down and not cry.'

Sam didn't become any less resilient moving to a different hospital. Understandably, she had difficulty coping with her new environment. Each one of us has a breaking point, when we feel like we can't go on. Many staff are already covering extra shifts and putting up with toxic working relationships.

How much more are they able to take, and are they expected to take? Resilience training, for me, isn't about teaching staff how to maintain their mental wellbeing in a healthcare system. I worry that it's training them to tolerate a deeply broken system.

Burnout

Everyone experiences stress. But when does a 'normal' amount of stress spill over into something else, which can render staff physically or psychologically unwell?

Burnout syndrome is defined as a chronic negative work-related psychological state, composed of three elements, which are:

1. High emotional exhaustion (referring to the physical/emotional overloads, or depletion of emotional resources);
2. High depersonalisation or lacking empathy with patients;
3. Low personal accomplishment, which is characterised by a negative work attitude towards work and low self-esteem due to unrewarding situations, which negatively impacts professional performance.[1]

In my experience, human-to-human connection is what staff find most nurturing and patients find so comforting. Yet when care becomes depersonalised, staff are starved of the very thing that nourishes them.

Jude, a midwife, discusses how being burnt out felt for her.

'When I look back now, I can see that what I was experiencing was burnout. Initially, I became tearful

over anything; it was more than just being sensitive. I then became emotionally exhausted, which was very physical, and I experienced 'unexplained' pains in my body. I began to dread going to work, and it took all the energy I had to get myself there. When I was on shift, I just couldn't focus on anything. I was supporting a mum during labour who was very anxious. Usually, I would've been calm, gentle, and reassuring towards her, but I felt nothing. I thought there was something seriously wrong with me. I took some time off work, and I began to recover and connect with those around me again.'

As well as significantly affecting an individual's wellbeing and quality of life, burnout can also have detrimental implications for the organisation involved by increasing absenteeism[2] and reducing service quality,[3] compromising patient safety.

Although many healthcare professionals are at risk of burnout, the characteristics of maternity professionals distinguish them from other staff working within the healthcare system. Many economic, organisational and professional factors, like professional shortages and poor working conditions, compromise the wellbeing of the maternity workforce.[4] This is further compounded by the significant emotional strain placed on them by potential complications, which can endanger the lives of mother and child.[5] Also, there is a high prevalence (25–35%) of anxiety and post-traumatic stress disorder in maternity staff,[6] making them potentially vulnerable to experiencing burnout. The highest rates of burnout are in newly qualified midwives[7] and trainee doctors working in obstetrics and gynaecology.[8] Furthermore, these medics are also at higher risk of experiencing anxiety, depression, suicidal thoughts, and substance misuse.

This is the next generation of maternity staff. Understanding why they are most affected and how to mitigate burnout is imperative if we are to retain the workforce and have safe, nurturing, and sustainable maternity services. Students on placement in maternity units can be a vital resource for more established staff and leaders to learn from. They come into practice after many hours of reading and academic work, so are in prime position to hold a mirror up to the environment they see. This is an invaluable asset to capture and be able to learn from to improve maternity for all who are in it. Improving the working conditions of maternity staff has been identified as essential to optimise their wellbeing. Furthermore, openness to communication, empathy, and individuals believing in their ability and skills to carry out their role (self-efficacy) have been identified as protective factors against burnout.[9,10]

Moral injury

Healthcare workers usually enter their profession to provide the best possible care, irrespective of a patient's gender, age, and condition. This desire is both their moral code and often their professional values. However, what if lack of resources, organisational issues, and toxic working cultures prevent staff from delivering the care they have been trained to provide? When this happens, their moral code can be shattered by making decisions that conflict with their professional values. The depths of their moral pain, which also signifies their humanity, indicate the degree to which their professional values have been violated.[11] Some staff have shared their experience of working for many years in a maternity system which has pulled them in too many directions. Before Covid-19 hit, there was already increasing recognition that healthcare professionals were experiencing moral distress, potentially leading to moral injury.[12]

During the pandemic, partners were unable to attend antenatal appointments and offer support throughout labour, and many staff were redeployed to other areas of healthcare. A report by Make Birth Better[13] found that many maternity staff felt heartbroken not to be able to provide the care to women they were trained to deliver, which increases the risk of moral injuries and trauma-related symptoms.[14] Some disclosed that their mental wellbeing had been negatively affected, and others explained how they felt traumatised. One midwife shared that she had *never wanted to leave the profession more*, and another said:

> *It's difficult to be able to provide the care that I came into the profession to provide. I spend a lot of time apologising for the changes to services. I feel like Covid-19 has sadly overshadowed the beauty and wonder of birth and autonomy of the woman.*

Many staff who shared decision-making felt supported by their colleagues and team. These factors appeared to mitigate the potential impact of moral injuries significantly.

Moral injury is defined as the psychological distress resulting from actions, or lack of them, which violate an individual's moral or ethical code.[15] Often the individual feels shame and guilt because they have not been able to right the wrong committed, alongside negative thoughts about oneself/others,[16] which are also symptoms of post-traumatic stress disorder (PTSD).[17] Although the moral injury is not a mental illness, exposure and the meaning of the events can lead to mental health difficulties like PTSD, suicidal ideation, depression, and anxiety.[15,16]

Currently, little is known about what interventions might

help to treat those affected by moral injuries. However, research is underway to get a better understanding of what might help. Many events and situations can lead to staff feeling morally distressed and injured. It is well known that social support can have a positive effect on psychological distress. However, when shame is a core feeling within that distress, social contact is usually avoided, isolating that individual further.[15] From my own experiences of supporting staff impacted by this, teaching them how to forgive themselves and foster self-compassion is crucial in helping them heal their broken spirit.

Stress response and anxiety

From time to time, we all feel anxious. In fact, at moments of stress, it can have positive benefits: it acts as an internal alarm to prompt action to prevent the worst scenario from happening. Like many mental health symptoms, how an individual experiences them varies from person to person. There are times when these feelings become more permanent and adversely impact an individual's mental wellbeing and quality of life. This differs from a typical stress-response, which passes.

When we encounter a perceived threat, a part of our brain, called the hypothalamus, triggers an alarm system in our body. A combination of hormonal and nerve signals are sent to our adrenal glands to release a surge of hormones (adrenaline and cortisol) to prepare us to manage the perceived threat. The adrenaline will increase our heartrate and blood pressure, enhancing our energy levels. Cortisol increases glucose in our bloodstream, to fuel the brain: it is like a superpower for the stress response. It acts to limit functions in our body that aren't essential to the fight-flight situation and supports the brain to think more clearly, which is needed at times of danger. Most of the time, when the stressful situation has passed, the stressful feelings (pounding heart, feeling jumpy, racing thoughts) tend to subside.

In the case of persistent feelings of stress, the internal alarm system can be triggered by anything (a smell, a situation, a place, a person, a noise), and it reacts as if it is a real threat when in fact it is a threat the individual *perceives* as dangerous. Anxiety is like the stress response going into overdrive. Often, a natural reaction to anxiety is to try and assert control and reduce fear. Control might feel like a temporary solution. However, working in maternity services can be unpredictable, and control becomes redundant in these situations as a coping strategy for anxiety.

In the case of midwives, evidence has suggested that younger, recently qualified midwives are at risk of personal burnout and experiencing heightened symptoms of anxiety and depression.[18] One potential explanation for this is that there is a mismatch between newly qualified midwives' ideals of midwifery work and the reality of working in maternity care.[19] However, as 'continuity of carer' models increase across the UK, this mismatch may begin to be addressed.

Experiencing anxiety symptoms can feel difficult, particularly because of the presence of thoughts that might be very loud in your mind. It is worth remembering that *thoughts are not facts, and feelings come and go*. Our minds can't predict the future, and they can't read other people's minds, even though they can sometimes do a great job of convincing us they can.

Psychological trauma

The majority of births have a positive outcome. However, in some cases, care does not go as expected, and so there might be a risk of severe injury or death for a mother or a baby. This can be a potentially traumatic experience for all involved, including staff. Listening to or witnessing traumatic perinatal events can create psychological distress in staff and lead to secondary traumatic stress (STS), which is the stress resulting from helping or wanting to help a traumatised or suffering person.[20]

The symptoms of STS are similar to PTSD and can include:[21]

- Increased negative arousal
- Intrusive thoughts/images of another's critical experiences
- Difficulty separating work from personal life
- Lowered frustration tolerance
- High outbursts of anger or rage
- Dread of working with specific individuals
- Depression
- Ineffective or self-destructive self-soothing behaviours
- Hypervigilance
- Decreased feelings of work competence
- A diminished sense of purpose/enjoyment with career
- Lowered functioning in non-professional situations
- Loss of hope

Although labelling mental health conditions can be helpful for individuals by informing them about what symptoms to look out for, the labels are primarily for clinicians so they can categorise and understand how people are presenting with mental health issues. However, people experience trauma symptoms differently, and staff can have trauma-related symptoms but never meet the diagnostic criteria. Don't let the fact that you don't 'tick all the boxes', or have a diagnosed named condition, allow your experiences to be squashed, denied, or undermined by others.

Unlike burnout, which develops gradually, the symptoms of STS can develop quickly and without much warning. Some staff may have risk factors that potentially increase their susceptibility to STS.

For example, each person comes to work with their own personal history of childhood, schooling, familial and relationship experiences. These will have shaped the person they have become and might have influenced their choice of profession. It is nigh on impossible to 'choose' which parts of yourself you bring to work and which parts are temporarily closed away. Given that the majority of information we process is at a subconscious level (without us knowing), it is likely that feelings will be brought to the fore at times during our career. We might not understand why we respond to a particular person, situation, or place in a particular way (this is called a trigger).

Sometimes this might not be particularly problematic and may be managed by an individual in a relatively straightforward way. However, past experiences as children and adults can predispose us to experience situations at work as destabilising and even traumatic, as highlighted below.

'The clinic started in the usual way, busy, rushed, and the waiting room filled up with women. I like the "buzz" of clinic, everyone knows what they need to do, and we all pull together to get on with it, like a well-oiled machine. I was on to my fifth appointment of the day, congratulating a couple on their long-awaited pregnancy news. I watched tears of joy fall down their cheeks and the tender look they shared with one another. My smile was fixed; I had said and done all the right things.

What they couldn't see, nor should they, was that inside, my heart wasn't just breaking. It was shattered *into a million pieces. Last week, I had been the patient who sat on the other side of the consultant's table. My husband and I, too, had shared tears of complete devastation and heartache that we would never have any children of our own.*

I knew how to be what I needed to be at work. What I hadn't learned at that time was how I needed to protect my own heart when the very job I loved triggered my fertility trauma.'

Anonymous, obstetrician and gynaecologist

For this obstetrician, her previous unresolved trauma activated her psychological distress and trauma symptoms when she encountered a similar work-related situation. Without seeking support to manage this, particularly when at work, being repeatedly exposed to similar triggers and subsequent distress could undoubtedly compromise her wellbeing further.

Another risk factor for developing STS is having experienced some kind of previous traumatic event.[20] Given that over one million people work for the NHS, it is likely that many of them will have experienced adverse and potentially traumatising events in their life. These will have been processed (or not) and will manifest differently in each person. The 'wounded healer', described by Carl Jung (when discussing a psychotherapist), highlighted that our own 'wounds' are often healed by attempting to heal others. Thus, many maternity staff might enter the profession to heal their trauma and possibly prevent others from being traumatised. However, when working in a maternity system they may sometimes feel unable to prevent trauma to those they are there to help. This can compound their distress further.

Reaching in

Mental health campaigns, public health messaging and social media bombard us with the message that if we're struggling with our mental health, we should reach out to others for support. I wholeheartedly support people doing this, but I think there's a big part of the conversation that's missing. Reaching out can be incredibly difficult for many people. I think we also need to discuss how to support *reaching in* – routinely checking on ourselves, our friends, family and other acquaintances.

We all experience mental health problems, and at times will suffer to a lesser or greater degree. It isn't always the person who is withdrawn, tearful, or low in mood who is struggling, because mental health has many faces. Someone who turns up to work each day, has a smile on their face, and looks like they're carrying on as usual, might still be grappling with difficult thoughts and feelings. So, rather than trying to differentiate between those who might need more support, we need to shift our mind-set and check in with those we come into contact with on a regular basis. Undoubtedly, many of us will be doing this already.

However, as our world has become more digital and online, some people are lacking a sense of physical community and feel isolated and as if they don't belong. The pandemic hasn't helped as we have been actively forced to withdraw from others, which will have compounded feelings of isolation and loneliness. Reaching out for support is complex and multifaceted. It involves taking a risk, in that we might not know how the other person will respond and if they will support us. Also, if layers of guilt, shame, stigma and other barriers are present, seeking support won't just feel tricky to do: it will feel like an enormous mountain to climb. We might also have a narrative that we've internalised about what it means to ask for help, which again hinders us. When people are struggling, they don't always know what they need, so identifying where to go can feel overwhelming.

When we become physically unwell, our body does a great job of alerting us through pain or discomfort, in an attempt to get us to slow down and tend to ourselves. However, when our mind gives us signals that we are in mental pain, feeling overwhelmed, low in mood or anxious, we can put mechanisms in place to dampen the symptoms, to block them out and detach, such as consuming alcohol or drugs, or telling ourselves (and others) that we're 'fine'. Reaching in to ourselves relies on connecting to a part of ourselves that is vulnerable and in pain. For many this is not safe or something they are willing or feel able to do, and it may feel strange and uncomfortable.

Reaching in to our colleagues, and those we support, isn't about absorbing their difficulties, stresses, or problems – rather, it's about connecting with them to say: 'I see you, I'm here for you, and you matter'. The smallest of actions we show to others can be embedded into their psyche as 'I am valued'. These are some suggestions meant to inspire you to begin creating your own:

- Rather than saying 'how are you?' as a greeting, ask it in a meaningful way, once, twice, three times, and make space and time to listen to the answer.
- Checking in with someone by text.
- Making a colleague a drink.
- Seeking out a colleague and acknowledging their contribution to the team.
- Normalising that working in maternity is challenging and difficult at times.
- Sending someone a card in the post.

Often when staff share with me the challenges of *reaching in* it isn't because they don't want to be a supportive colleague. Usually, they too are feeling overwhelmed, overstretched and unable to make space in their heads and hearts for someone else. It's symptomatic of compassion fatigue and burnout. I think it's worth remembering that we don't have to be effused with feelings of love and kindness to show these to others. If we prioritise caring for ourselves and our colleagues, and actively look for opportunities to *reach in* and practice these acts, we will all feel more supported.

Over the years, there have been some ground-breaking technological advances in maternity care. But prioritising the wellbeing of the workforce has been slower to catch on as an idea. As part of their training, maternity professionals need to be taught about their potential vulnerability to working in maternity care, including the signs and symptoms of conditions such as STS, and stress-related coping behaviours, like numbing responses. Also, they need to know how to identify these in colleagues, and ways to respond. Peer support, setting professional boundaries, and creating potential responses to challenging scenarios at work, could also prove helpful in shielding against the impact of working in an emotionally intense environment. We can't assume that people will *reach out* if they need support. Erring on the side of caution, and *reaching in* to ourselves and colleagues, can have a long-standing and potentially life-changing impact on some people. There are further suggestions in Chapter 5 about some ways to optimise mental wellbeing on an organisational, team, and individual level.

2

WORKING IN A
TRAUMATISED SYSTEM

The emotional cost of caring

Most healthcare professionals enter their profession to provide the best possible care, irrespective of the patient's gender, age, and condition. As discussed, this is their moral code and often their professional values. However, many work in a system that doesn't allow this code to be practised. Even before they have finished training, or early in their careers, many consider moving to another job, or worst still, leaving their profession. The gruelling off-duty rotas, toxic culture, sleep deprivation, lack of support, or high stress levels become unsustainable.

This distinct culture is one in which, according to Dr Robin Youngson, founder of Hearts in Healthcare and author of *Time to Care: How to Love Your Patients and Your Job*[1], '*the rules are clear: put your head down, complete your tasks as quickly as possible, get the paperwork done, and move onto the next patient.*' In such a culture there is little recognition of the emotional impact of the job on staff, who require a supportive, psychologically safe environment. The high levels of burnout are often met with surprise. When staff are abused, humiliated, and dehumanised, we expect that they will still show compassion, kindness, and empathy to those in their care. Emotional detachment, therefore, isn't a conscious choice: it's a necessity to survive.

Renée Fox, a medical sociologist at the University of Pennsylvania, said, *'Doctors' anguish seems to come from violating every day what they know they ought to be doing. The pain is from the degree to which they still espouse values but can't live up to them'.* This is what I bear witness to in those staff who come to see me for support. They are part of an organisation where their work-related values are compromised, and their moral code is shattered. Apart from the distress this causes, the intensity of guilt and shame many experience can be overwhelming. Many have shared with me times when they have rushed a patient, spoken sharply, been rude, avoided human connection with the person in their care, walked away when a mother became distressed or made a gross error of judgement. Some of these actions were intentional, and others were not. They are often symptoms that staff need support and care. Some might feel more equipped to shake these experiences off, and perhaps in the short term feel they were unaffected. However, it is severely emotionally wounding for others. Each instance of providing or witnessing poor care has an impact, to the point where it becomes unbearable. This is when many feel their mental wellbeing is becoming compromised.

Although many staff feel powerless to change the system, having fulfilling interactions with those they support during their pregnancy journey, in birth, and postnatally can be healing. Some of these exchanges could be:

- introducing yourself
- having a gentle tone of voice

- respecting and promoting choice
- making eye contact
- smiling
- gentle touch (with consent)

Learning to stay connected in the relationship with the mother, no matter how brief the encounter, is nurturing and protective for both staff and patient.

The role of fear in maternity

'I got to the stage where I was having panic attacks before my shift started. I was frozen in the car. The thought of going back on the ward not only filled me with worry, but I was also terrified I would bump into him. That he would be there, watching my work, scrutinising everything I did, and I couldn't get away, I was trapped, having to finish my shift, make pretty big decisions for patients. It was almost inevitable I was going to make a mistake. I prayed it wouldn't be to the detriment of a patient or her baby.'

Anonymous, obstetrician who experienced
bullying by a consultant colleague

Fear has many faces, and no one is immune from it. This obstetrician's fears lay in a range of areas that many staff report harms their mental wellbeing: being bullied, watched, criticised, and potentially causing harm to a patient and her baby. It isn't always so obvious, like the 'freezing' experienced by this obstetrician. However, it is essential to know what the signs are when you are experiencing fear and how this might present when at work, mainly because fear can alter our perception and behaviour in situations.

Our brains are excellent at making associations and are hardwired to protect us. Most of the time they do a pretty good job, but sometimes they can go into overdrive. For example, imagine that while supporting a woman during birth, the clinician or midwife missed something vital. When they recognised this, they had a surge of adrenaline (fear response), which propelled them to act, and the outcome of the birth was positive for all involved. At that moment, because of that experience, the neurons in their brain will have a changed pattern,[2] potentially setting them up to feel fearful when they're in a similar 'near miss' situation in the future. Where do they turn to discuss what has just happened, what led to the 'near miss', to soothe themselves and explore how they might be feeling about it?

By bringing this to their team, they're providing a learning opportunity for everyone and also, crucially, accessing support (if needed) for themselves. In the absence of this, they might begin to feel less confident, spend more time documenting the decisions they have made and begin to practise more defensively.

In jobs that reward individuals with speed and accuracy, like factory staff on an assembly line, fear was once viewed as a motivator to ensure productivity. However, working in maternity requires immense skill in building relationships, rapport, and trust with others, sometimes in chaotic and emotionally intense situations. For maternity staff to do this effectively, they need to feel physically and psychologically safe at work. That sounds like a pretty essential requirement, but we know this is absent in many teams and organisations.

The fears of 739 staff, mostly midwives, were analysed to reveal the top eight fears they experienced at work.[3] These were:

1. Death of a baby
2. Missing something that causes harm
3. Obstetric emergency
4. Maternal death
5. Being watched or criticised
6. Being the cause of a negative birth experience
7. Dealing with the unknown and not being prepared
8. Losing my passion and confidence in normal birth

Midwives indicated that defensive practice had been born from a need to protect themselves from liability and their fears relating to litigation. For some, their fear of litigation has increased and has negatively impacted the normal birth process, as midwives prioritise their need for self-protection.

I have never met anyone working in maternity services who entered their career to cause harm to others, whether colleagues or mothers. However, in the UK, although maternity cases equated to only 10% of the overall clinical negligence claims in 2018–19, they accounted for 50% of the total value of claims received by NHS Resolution, totalling £2.5 billion.[4] The high cost is because injury at birth for a baby or mother can have catastrophic effects over a lifetime.[5] Unsurprisingly, fear of litigation is a genuine concern for many maternity staff.

A lawyer colleague and I run workshops for maternity staff called 'Saying Sorry Doesn't Mean Litigation'. What I've learned over the years is that staff involved in an adverse event usually want to express regret about what happened and apologise to the family involved for any shortcomings in their treatment. In my experience, families want this too. However, this is difficult for staff to do, as many have been 'warned' by their organisation to have no contact with the family. This helps no one.

Being involved in a serious incident requiring investigation (SIRI), not being able to humanely connect with those impacted, and being suspended often has a profound psychological impact on the staff involved. Before an incident, it is likely that the mental wellbeing of maternity staff will have been compromised and that the event further compounds those existing feelings. A study of over 3,000 obstetricians and gynaecologists found that 36% met the criteria for burnout and were six times more like to experience suicidal thoughts, four times more likely to report depression, and three times more likely to report anxiety, irritability, and anger. Those with burnout were four times more likely to practise defensively, meaning they might avoid complex cases or procedures, over-prescribe medications, carry out more investigations or procedures than necessary for fear of making a mistake, or miss a diagnosis.[6]

For some staff, over time, these difficult feelings can diminish. However, others are left finding it hard to function. Most NHS Trusts offer a formal debriefing to those involved to begin to emotionally process the traumatic event and build resilience to further events. However, some staff want access to counselling, and in many cases this is not available.[7] The Confidential Enquiry into Maternal and Child Health 2000–2002[8] advised that staff involved in a maternal death should be offered supportive counselling. However, in the absence of formal and informal support, some evidence has found that distressed midwives will seek support from women using maternity services.[9] This is symptomatic of staff desperately needing help and their difficulty containing their psychological distress in the workplace. One mum shared how 'they need to be supported from within. They can't be reliant on the birthing mothers to hold their hands and pat them on the back.'[9]

It is essential to know that everyone's ability to cope with the effects of significant stress or trauma differs, and having access to support will facilitate recovery.[10] These experiences can undoubtedly leave their mark on the professionals involved. Some are haunted by these events throughout their careers and carry the associated weight of shame and guilt. To psychologically and professionally protect themselves, they might begin to practise defensively, perform medically unjustified caesarean sections[11,12] and emotionally detach from patients.

Employers have a duty of care to ensure staff are fit to work. Sadly, despite recommendations by governing bodies and reports, I continue to receive emails and self-referrals from staff who feel isolated, distressed, and unsupported by their organisation. This needs to change if we are to create a psychologically healthy workforce where staff are valued and nurtured.

Psychological safety: can we be attached to a healthcare system?

Psychology undergraduates learn about the fundamental importance of something called attachment. According to this approach, attachment runs through every thread of a relationship. As psychologists, we are fine-tuned to assess and look out for attachment in those we treat because it has such a significant impact on how relationships are formed and how individuals respond in return. There are four different attachment styles, but I only want to mention two: secure and ambivalent attachment. If a person is securely attached to their caregiver, they feel protected, safe, and they know they can depend on them. So, in adult relationships, they feel secure, and even when there is disharmony, they don't feel abandoned or that the relationship is at risk of breaking down. Ambivalent attachment is when someone learns that their caregiver is unreliable. They might have been neglectful, unavailable, or inconsistent, and the individual understands that they can't depend on any relationship. So, as an adult, they might be mistrustful of others and seek proof of their love. Understanding how attached to the healthcare system staff are could help them know how they respond to it.

For example, let's consider that the healthcare system is the 'caregiver'. Currently, some staff might feel ambivalently attached because sometimes their Trust puts on a wellbeing day, offers them free yoga, encourages them to stay hydrated, and momentarily they might feel valued. However, suppose that most of the time their experience is that the organisation overworks them. Resources are cut, and staff are not supported when they need it the most, despite the lip-service to 'wellbeing'. It is likely they will become mistrustful and won't feel valued or believe that their Trust has their best interests at heart. Conversely, if staff worked in Trusts where they were 'securely attached', it would mean they would feel safe, valued, and supported, even when times became tough or something went wrong.

A midwife shares the following story:

'I still feel haunted by that day. Being involved in the death of a baby goes entirely against what I came into this profession to do. And yet, I missed the signs. I was tired, we were seriously short-staffed, and I didn't listen to the mum when she shared her concerns with me. I didn't have time.

I wept with the family when I passed them their baby. At that moment, I knew that I had a part to play in their baby's death. I was deeply sorry, and I said so.

After this, I went on to deliver two more healthy babies and finished my shift. The following day I received a call from my senior manager to say I was suspended while the investigation took place. The next months were a blur.

I eventually returned to work, and I felt like a criminal. The shame and guilt that I felt were unbearable. Colleagues I had worked with for over 20 years were told not to speak to me by my manager. I was an outcast.

After 22 years working in midwifery, I left the profession, and it utterly shattered my world and broke my heart.'

This midwife was not only involved in a traumatic event, and experienced the moral injury of it, but she was cruelly neglected by her seniors and rejected by her peers. It is likely she was not emotionally ready to return to work. Crucially, the environment she worked in and was returning to was psychologically unsafe. Amy Edmondson at Harvard defines psychological safety in the team context as '*a belief that one will not be punished or humiliated for speaking up with ideas, questions, concerns, or mistakes, and that the team is safe for interpersonal risk-taking.*' [13]

Taking a risk and speaking out when staff don't know what the outcome will be takes courage and vulnerability. If you work in a team where someone shares something and everyone responds with openness and respect, it's more likely you will feel safe to expose your vulnerability or admit a mistake. However, if fear of being belittled and judged is something you've observed as a weapon to keep people in check, self-protection will feel paramount. Many people hold the view that vulnerability is a weakness. Brené Brown explains that vulnerability is '*uncertainty, risk and emotional* exposure. It is the source of hope, empathy, accountability, and authenticity'. To be vulnerable is rarely weak. Some of the examples of vulnerability I have observed in maternity care include:

- A student midwife sharing with her team how emotional she had found her day.
- An obstetrician asking for forgiveness from a family when care did not go as expected.
- A junior doctor speaking out about feeling exhausted and needing to rest.
- A ward manager kindly telling her senior that all staff would have their breaks.
- An anaesthetist listening to a distressed mum and providing reassurance.
- The consultant obstetrician asking her colleague if she was okay.
- The clinical lead spending time openly listening to the difficult feedback her colleagues shared about a decision she had made.

To me, none of these are acts of weakness, rather the opposite. To show up, connect with another person, accept accountability, and speak the truth, takes courage, risk, and some willingness to feel uncomfortable when the outcome is unknown.

Imagine if the midwife who shared her experience had worked in a team where psychological safety was an integral part of how they functioned, where her colleagues and the organisation reached out and asked, 'What happened?' rather than 'Who did it?'. What if, when she returned to work, she was met with respect and support, rather than rejection and judgement?

For real change to happen, psychological safety needs to be adopted from the bottom up (individual) and the top down (culture). It's not one or the other; both are essential. Dan Radecki and Leonie Hull from the Academy of Brain Based Leadership[14] describe psychologically safe cultures as ones which 'value and promote psychological safety as a cultural standard. They protect psychological safety through policy, process, and practice, and are accountable to the psychological safety standards and expectations'. A leader who is present, understanding, can empathise with staff, and help the other person (emotionally or practically) will positively contribute to creating a psychologically safe culture.[15]

Each individual working in maternity can foster the right conditions to harness nurture and compassion. These do not necessarily need to be large acts of grandeur. Rather they will often be small acts of kindness and connection with another person. For example, when you see a colleague who is stressed, what is your usual reaction? Do you give them a knowing smile as you pass, to say, 'I see you, I relate to the stress you're under', do you make them a cup of tea, offer to help in some way, or do you put your head down and walk on, hoping they don't notice you? Perhaps you feel stressed yourself and as though you don't have time to shoulder anyone else's burdens.

Connecting with another person is a choice. It doesn't have to be time-consuming; it is *how* we connect that makes a difference. We are not emotional islands. We are primarily social creatures. As Thomas Sy, assistant professor at California State University Long Beach, reports, 'if I want to be part of this group, I will think and act and behave – and in this case, feel – like the rest of my group members'. Therefore, as individuals, we can commit to conveying acts of kindness and compassion, mainly because emotions and our responses can be contagious to others. It hard not to smile back at someone who smiles at us; we're wired to be social.

Edmondson[13] created a robust measure to assess psychologically safety in teams by asking the following:

1. If you make a mistake on this team, it is often held against you –
2. Members of this team are able to bring up problems and tough issues +
3. People on this team sometimes reject others for being different –
4. It is safe to take a risk on this team +
5. It is difficult to ask other members of this team for help –
6. No one on this team would deliberately act in a way that undermines my efforts +
7. Working with members of this team, my unique skills and talents are valued and utilised +

If you answer yes to all the questions marked by a + sign and no to those marked with a – sign, you are probably working in a team with high levels of psychological safety. This is important because those working in a psychologically safe environment are more likely to feel appreciated, valued, able to take a risk to be vulnerable, admit mistakes, and support their colleagues.

At Make Birth Better[16] we developed the conceptual model below. This was based on several workshops with maternity staff, families, policymakers, and academics about ways to prevent birth trauma and reduce its impact on all involved in the birthing process.

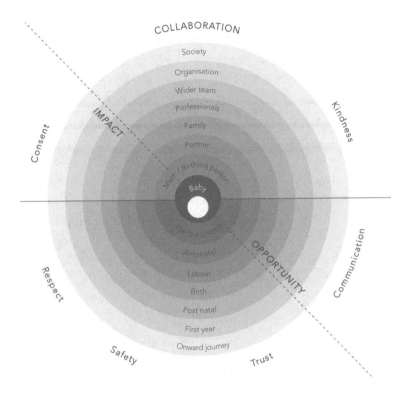

The Make Birth Better Model

The values surrounding the circle of collaboration, kindness, communication, trust, safety, respect, and consent are vital behaviours that need to be applied by the organisation to the wider team and professionals, which will positively impact mothers and their partners.

Psychological safety is essential to ensure staff perform at their best, although it's not the only ingredient required. The role of leadership is pivotal, not only to create psychological safe cultures, learning opportunities and prevent avoidable errors, but also to *'allow more mental space for the medical team to focus on the patient, which is currently one of the weakest links in health care, and that's a good thing. After all, as Hippocrates observed a few millennia* ago, "It is far more important to know what person has the disease than what disease the person has,'" according to Roel van der Heijdeis, a partner at the Patient-Centered Care Association in The Netherlands, and Dirk Deichmann, who is an associate professor at Erasmus University's Rotterdam School of Management.

Working in maternity care is a physically and emotionally demanding job. However, it doesn't have to be one where staff and patients are left to navigate an unsafe healthcare system. In a world where medical error is a leading cause of death, the emotional impact on staff wellbeing cannot be underestimated. This can also be compounded by an overstretched workforce, compromised mental wellbeing, understaffing, and emotional exhaustion. Understanding yourself, your triggers, and how you manage these is the first step in supporting your wellbeing. It might help individual staff stay connected with themselves and not become detached in response to difficulties. Having team members that are open, transparent, and kind will normalise the emotional load of working in maternity care. This, in turn, will help staff feel safe to be vulnerable and step into courage when needed. Again, connecting with the other person is vital; individuals can choose to engage in small acts of kindness and compassion. Having an organisation that values psychological safety and has measures implemented to reflect this will contribute to staff feeling valued for their work and help them feel nurtured and cared for. Therefore, the leadership of the organisation is crucial to ensuring this happens.

Key messages

- Fear is prevalent in maternity staff and impacts negatively on their wellbeing.
- Understanding what triggers work-related fears and how staff respond to these is the first step in learning a different way to manage them.
- Connection is critical: with yourself, your colleagues, and those you care for.
- Taking a risk to be vulnerable takes courage and strength.
- Individual staff can influence the culture of the team and the organisation they work in.
- Choosing to be kind and compassionate to colleagues can be contagious.

PERSON-CENTRED AND COMPASSIONATE LEADERSHIP

Karen Ledger

'Yesterday I was clever, so I wanted to change the world.
Today I am wise, so I am changing myself.'

Rumi

Good leadership can make a world of difference to an organisation and its staff by ensuring they have a clear pathway to carry out their job well. For leaders and the people in the organisation, positive and effective relationships are a win-win for all. Leaders develop an organisation's culture and oversee the structure. For example, they provide sufficient staffing levels and highly trained managers who can then ensure the right equipment, tuition, and policies are in place to enable maternity staff to practise competently and safely. Conversely, poor leadership can have a devastating effect on an organisation's culture and lead to toxic environments where there are high levels of stress, absenteeism, and poor retention of staff.

As a person-centred executive coach, psychotherapist, trainer, and supervisor, I have worked with many senior leaders from the NHS. I understand the need for effective leadership in the NHS. My working life began in the 1970s in the NHS as a nurse; I then became a leader in local authority services for the elderly, culminating as a specialist social worker and NHS training consultant in HIV and sexual health in the mid-1990s. I then began my independent practice as a trainer, OD consultant, therapist, and expert witness for people who have catastrophic injuries, including medical negligence. Approximately 15 to 20 years ago I incorporated executive coaching into my practice, and since that time I have mostly worked with leaders from the NHS. Sadly, a number of these sought coaching because of their poor experiences. I have learned from my own and others' experiences why positive and practical leadership matters.

I bring together person-centred theory and compassionate leadership because I can see how they can complement and work together to support leaders to be fully present and conscious. I recognise the importance of acknowledging the pockets of the NHS that are working and are well-led. I hope that bringing two evidence-based approaches together will inspire you and the leader in you to make the NHS world a better place for women and staff.

Person-centred and compassionate leadership

Carl Rogers developed person-centred theory/philosophy in 1940 as a theory for psychotherapy. It has continued to be developed by Rogers and others since then. Many of the theories for coaching have a background in psychotherapy approaches, for example gestalt, transactional analysis, and relational coaching. I have adapted the person-centred theory for leadership.

Rogers believed that favourable environmental conditions would lead to human growth and the ability to reach full potential. Fundamental to the theory are six conditions which he described as necessary and sufficient. I have adapted these conditions to offer a proposal for leadership:

1. *Two persons are in psychological contact* – this could be a leader and a group of people or individuals of the team. Therefore, all relevant and relational persons are in contact for this condition to be working.

2. *The first person (staff member) is in a state of incongruence, being vulnerable or anxious* – this will inevitably be happening for individuals or groups in any organisation.

3. *The second person (the leader) is congruent.* That is a state of genuineness, transparency, and integration. A form of being authentic and without façade – being fully in touch with our experience, a self-awareness that is perceived as trustworthy. I prefer to describe congruence as being available for the relationship with the people they are leading.

4. *The leader experiences unconditional positive regard for the staff they are serving* – this is where compassionate leadership and the person-centred approach are at one. Rogers believed that for people to grow and fulfil their potential, they must be valued as themselves. Genuine care and acceptance that each human being is of equal value.

5. *That the leader is experiencing an empathic understanding of the individual's or team's internal frame of reference* – Rogers described empathy as 'To sense the client's [person's] world as if it were your own but without losing the "as if" quality – this is empathy'.[1] The experiencing of an accurate understanding of another's awareness and experience, i.e., walking in another's shoes as if they were our own to understand the person's meaning, while not losing the 'as if' quality and remaining a

separate being. This condition also meets compassionate leadership, and they seem to me to be part of the same family.

6. That staff perceives, at least to a minimal degree, conditions 4 and 5, the unconditional positive regard of the leader for her/him/them.[*]

The components in compassionate leadership are not dissimilar to the conditions as laid out above. I suggest that they are dove-tailed together to work in harmony and for all the person-centred conditions and compassionate components to be activated within the context of the relationship. For example:

- *Attending*: noticing of a person or persons' suffering. This is similar to being in psychological contact, condition one and two, that the person is in a state of anxiety or vulnerability.
- *Understanding*: an appraisal of the cause and resources to cope and help. The following two components fit with condition six of empathic understanding, to sense the person's world as if it were the leader's own.
- *Empathising*: a felt response to the other's distress. Person-centred condition two as explained above.
- *Helping*: taking thoughtful, intelligent action to relieve the other's suffering. This would fit with condition six, that staff, to at least a minimum degree, perceive unconditional positive regards and empathic understanding. [**]

---

[*] Adapted from Rogers' conditions necessary and sufficient for therapeutic personality change and in this instance necessary for relational leadership, 1957, 1959.[2]

[**] Modified from West and Chowla 2017, chapter 13, Atkins & Parker 2012.[3]

I consider that the person-centred six conditions and the compassionate components provide a structure to support the formulation of a relationship in a leadership context. This structure is relevant to provide a type of leadership model of practice.

While person-centred and compassionate leadership are theoretically simple and therefore accessible, their practice is not. In my experience, implementing them requires ongoing intentional practice, attention, and commitment. To be genuine and authentic usually means that we have to run the risk of personal exposure and vulnerability. However, if this is achieved, the rewards are immense, and we can gain from having much more fulfilling and engaging relationships at work and in our personal lives. This is because both person-centred and compassionate leadership are relational approaches and put the connection at the heart of leadership.

Three of the above conditions are known as the 'core conditions': congruence, unconditional positive regard, and empathy. Except for congruence, the two remaining states, unconditional positive regard and empathy are now in general use. Empathy is regularly used in health services, and I hear people describe it as 'walking or being in another's shoes'. This carries a risk of entanglement in someone's feelings or process without remaining separate, which might be experienced as confusing, blurring, or patronising for the person on the receiving end.

Empathy is to sense a person's feelings, whether it is anger, fear or confusion, or a positive feeling such as joy, while keeping a separateness without losing the 'as if' quality. To reiterate, we need to walk in another's shoes as if they are our own.

In my experience, empathy takes endless practice and constant attention and is not something we can just do. However, I appreciate that some people are more naturally attuned to empathy than others. I hear people describing interpersonal skills as 'soft skills'. This is often said in quite a disparaging way, as if they are not as essential and valuable as business development and financial skills, for example.

Over the years, I have heard leaders make the following comments about their leadership:

- I don't have the time to invest in people
- Being empathic does not work – it's too fluffy
- Being kind to staff will breed complacency
- They need managing closely, or they will make mistakes
- If you are too nice to staff, they take advantage of you
- I am not touchy-feely

All the above statements are myths because when staff are provided with reflective spaces, they can absorb and integrate their experience, which leads to them feeling more relaxed, confident, and content in their work. They will make fewer mistakes and feel free to be creative and make mistakes, so long as they feel respected and supported. Relational cultures breed psychological safety. Toxic and unsafe environments create stress and fear for staff, which takes more energy and is depleting.

In my view, the person-centred approach is based on tenderness and wholeheartedness, which requires leaders to have a high level of self-awareness to meet the relational demands. Person-centred and relational leadership pays attention to staff, and therefore implicit in the organisation is recognition that staff are the most critical resource.

The importance of self-awareness

Person-centred leadership starts with a focus on self, and an incisive leader may ask themselves questions similar to the below:

- Who am I?
- Why do I lead?
- What type of leader am I?
- Does this fit with the leader I want to be?
- What do I need to develop?

I became a leader in the 1980s to contribute to a system I knew was underrepresented in working within services for older people. It was not an altruistic move because it also served my need to move on from being a nurse, where I felt creatively stifled by an autocratic leadership system.

As a leader, I quickly saw how making small changes in the residential services for the elderly could make significant differences to clients and staff. For example, the introduction of an acting-up scheme (stepping into a more senior position) enabled care staff to find the leader in themselves.

Implicit in person-centred and compassionate leadership is wellbeing. If we begin by having empathy and transparency for ourselves, we can start to put those conditions in place for others. Self-discovery and awareness are the voyages of a lifetime. Having experienced almost 30 years of self-development work, I appreciate how rocky the self-discovery road can be. I also reap the vast liberating benefits of feeling more of who I am based on my understanding, rather than before when I was told by others about who I am. I feel more confident as a person and therefore in my roles as a woman, therapist, coach, mother, partner, and friend.

Self-awareness is about looking inwards and what I

refer to as internal inquiry or reflecting on your internal landscape. This takes conscious work, and developing self-awareness is never complete. We can always reveal more to ourselves about who we are. To begin this process, you could reflect on why you chose a career in maternity or as a leader.

Leaders who look for external fixes miss the essential internal work that goes into excellent and effective leadership. The external fixes may be described as, for example, change management, strategies, technical support, or policy. These approaches can support leadership and staff teams, but they are not enough in themselves. We are social beings and are nurtured by being connected to others.

Being aware of our strengths, developmental needs, personality, and biases, has a significant impact on how leaders behave and interact with others. In being self-aware, a leader can consciously influence the situation and the culture of the organisation. We cannot operate in the conditions of regard, empathy, and authenticity without self-awareness.

Being self-aware can lead to extraordinary leadership and is a prerequisite to being an effective leader. Self-awareness is not an easy process and requires self-compassion, kindness, and patience. The more we can accept the way we are, the more fluid and flexible we become, making us ready for change when needed.

Why being in the relationship matters

Without the relationship, we are in the wilderness. All communication takes place most effectively within a relationship. We can craft the most eloquent communication, but these messages will be lost in the absence of the relationship. The connection provides meaning to our communication and unification, sharing and supporting a common purpose of providing care to patients.

When we are out of the relationship, we ignore what the person is saying because we do not care enough. Therefore, if leaders are not engaged with their staff, both messages will be lost. It is short-sighted for any leader not to pay attention to the people and their welfare.

Regard, empathy, and genuineness are the conditions that can support leaders to form all-important working (and personal) relationships. I offer this philosophy as a model to work with, practise, and be fundamental to leadership. It is a straightforward model that takes commitment, discipline, practice, and skill. This cannot be overestimated in my experience.

An effective relationship provides a safe vessel for those necessary difficult and complex conversations. If the vessel is not sufficiently watertight and robust, it will leak and sink like any other container. If the relationship is adequate, it will hold conflict, challenge, and positive forces, such as success and joy. This, of course, does not mean it has to be a close, intimate relationship, only that it has to be sufficient and include respect, transparency, empathy, and regard.

Jess Read, Deputy Chief Midwifery Officer for England, shares her experience of providing compassionate leadership.

'I was fortunate to undertake my midwifery training at the British Hospital for Mothers and Babies in Woolwich, a small maternity hospital with a midwifery training school attached. My midwifery tutor was Sister Christine, one of the "Nursing Sisters of St John the Divine" whose previous faith communities became so well-known through the popular Call the Midwife series. I still have

my file of notes given out by Sister Christine during my 18-month training, and right at the very front of the file is the following quote:

> "A midwife must constantly put out effort to stay compassionate, open, and clear in her vision, for love and compassion are two of the most important tools of her trade."

I have no idea where that quote came from, but it has stayed with me and has proven to be so very true over the years. How much more so now as the NHS faces its greatest challenge of the global pandemic. Almost 37,000 midwives are employed in the UK and are responsible for facilitating care to ensure 640,500 safe births per year. I am aware of the profound impact this pandemic has had on the health and wellbeing of nurses and midwives.

Throughout my career, I have been privileged to develop others, individuals and teams and watch them thrive and flourish. When midwives are met with dignity and respect, I have seen that they are encouraged to work autonomously where they control their working lives and are valued for their vital and essential contribution; compassionate and safe cultures abound.

Every one of us has a responsibility to be kind and compassionate and to respect the dignity of our co-workers and the women and families we care for. Indeed, two of the six NHS values are Respect and Dignity, and Compassion. Wherever we work, and at every level, we can all positively impact the lives of others.

In my practice, I have a strong sense of the need to sustain inclusive, just, fair, and psychologically safe cultures; this requires proactive activity, reaching out to ensure equity, and role-modelling behaviours that promote diversity and support inclusivity. I aim to ensure that everyone I interact with feels valued, listened to, and can thrive.

I love this quote from Sheila Kitzinger:

"In all cultures, the midwife's place is on the threshold of life, where intense human emotions, fear, hope, longing, triumph, and incredible physical power enable a new human being to emerge. The midwife's vocation is unique."

Now more than ever, midwives need compassionate leadership to flourish and thrive, and every one of us has a part to play in achieving that.'

The importance of communication

Dialogue and conversation are how we stay connected. It helps us understand how we are, the quality of the relationships we have, and how the people that matter to us are. To promote and maintain connectedness in the NHS, there should be many formal and informal communication streams, where feedback can be given horizontally and vertically. This does not mean that leaders have relationships with everyone, but that there is an organisational interconnectedness. People are supported, and they know the direction the organisation is heading and their role in it. For example, staff at any level would know how to communicate openly with maternity leaders formally and informally, and opportunities would be created for this.

During the Covid pandemic, I have talked to NHS leaders and staff about how they can stay connected and support one another. During such periods as change management, a trauma in the service, or a crisis such as a pandemic, staff need extra care and more communication. It is therefore very relevant to provide additional thinking and feeling space and support. Debriefing sessions after trauma and time spent processing and reflecting are very important.

In addition, check-ins and check-outs at the beginning and end of the day for the staff can be extremely helpful. Some of the sessions have agendas, and others do not. One staff member had introduced a fun quiz to share social time for his NHS team working from home during the pandemic. More restorative supervision and reflective practice sessions have also been working for teams I have been involved with. The staff teamed with leaders who have introduced more communication streams report, on the whole, being emotionally intact. In contrast, those trying to work as they did before the pandemic largely report emotional and physical fatigue.

Sheena Byrom, OBE, reflects on her experience of compassionate leadership:

> 'I have had the most amazing and fulfilling career. I am a practising midwife of 40 plus years, now a midwifery consultant sharing my expertise (and learning too!) globally – and I own a business with my midwife daughter Anna in which we strive to support and nurture midwives and maternity workers through creative learning and development.
>
> It was the week after I had safely facilitated a water birth at home. I was so proud; the mother and family were ecstatically happy. I'd never seen a baby born in water before; it was 1993 and not commonplace at all. A wonderful head of midwifery supported me, and I gave the woman what she wanted. Sadly, my direct line manager didn't like me, and she made it obvious on many occasions. So early on Monday morning, I was

called to the manager's office. She had been on annual leave when the birth took place, and she wanted to speak to me "for feedback", she said. I was expecting her to ask about the event and congratulate me. Instead, she sat opposite me behind a desk and pointed to the pink hospital record containing the delivery details. With a straight face, she asked me why I hadn't given the Syntometrine (an injected drug to help the placenta to separate) immediately after the birth. These are the specifics of the care that I'm not able to debate here – needless to say, the mother wanted to wait until she left the pool before receiving the drug.

I was devasted by my manager's treatment, especially as I knew I had given exemplary care, and I was elated with the outcome. I started to cry. My manager didn't move or show any concern. She just sat quietly, observing my distress – no offer of tissues, no reaction. After a few minutes, I stood up and left. As I passed through the door, another community midwife was entering – she was our manager's favourite, the one she kept close by her side. Here I was, a grown woman with four children and a successful career – distressed by the actions of my superior. The incident was never mentioned again. This was not an isolated event but one which stirred a fire in me. And this particular manager was not the only one who treated me and others with contempt. It was a regular occurrence and something I thought I had to get used to but never did. I wouldn't accept this if I had to revisit that time, though I learned from each bullying episode – I vowed never to be a bully of others.

I didn't reflect on the concept of leadership until I became a midwifery manager myself years later – when I discovered that I missed the intimate connection with *the women and families I served during clinical work. This coincided with my study for a master's degree in which I delved into personality traits and various approaches to leadership. I also recognised that when I treated the midwives I was managing with the same care and attention as the women in my caseload as a clinical midwife, my job satisfaction improved and I felt happier with my position. The midwives and other maternity workers responded positively on the whole – I learned how to negotiate compassionately and later, as a consultant midwife, to provide authentic positive feedback and witness the difference it made. Nurturing and valuing my colleagues became a priority, and it still is. I have seen the impact this has, how services are safer and positive outcomes are maximised.*

I really must stress that my career has been heavily influenced by positive role models – leaders who challenged the status quo and inspired me to do the same. These individuals focused on the needs of those using our services as a priority, but we, as colleagues, were nurtured too and treated with respect. I was given opportunities to grow and develop and eventually became the head of midwifery, which was totally unexpected. My various leadership roles have given me the opportunity to influence the culture of a shift, a department, and an organisation. Mostly, I now understand that leaders can be and are at every level of the organisation – they just need the right environment to flourish.'

Person-centred leadership is more about being than doing. For example, it is about creating and developing relationships as a vehicle to enable people to get on with their jobs in a relaxed and harmonious environment without risk of judgment. This does not mean that negative and positive feedback will not be offered, or that disciplinary procedures will not be implemented when necessary.

I feel that during the process of a disciplinary procedure, the need to protect the relationship is more significant than ever. This then allows the disciplined person to be upset and angry without being ostracised by their leader while continuing to feel regarded and understood. During a disciplinary situation, the staff member might feel a range of emotions, which can threaten their ability to remain in the relationship. As a leader, working to maintain respect, value, and empathy in this context might also feel compromising at times. Therefore, having an awareness of what helps to stay in the relationship during emotionally intense and challenging situations will be advantageous; for staff, the leader, and ultimately the organisation.

How to respond when care does not go as expected

Hopefully, before this happens, relationships will be fully functioning, creating safety for staff and leaders alike, with communication flowing freely both ways. Leaders can then have an honest, frank, and challenging conversation about what led to events not going as expected and understanding this.

I provided coaching to someone recently who had made an error that led to her dismissal. She had made a wrong decision because she did not feel safe and supported by her leaders and could not, therefore, communicate her difficulties effectively and be supported to resolve them. She chose the wrong course of action and lost her position. Had she had strong leadership to support and guide her, it may have saved her employment.

In Chapter 2 we saw an example of a midwife who didn't

feel she had time to fully listen to the concerns of a mother, which had devastating consequences. If you think you do not have time, you are in a vulnerable place where mistakes can be made. This is the time to shout for help, because mothers, babies, and you are at risk. In a relational service, staff and leaders would jump to support rather than make dismissive responses such as 'we are all in the same boat'. When care falls below the expected standard, it is imperative to remove blame as this does not serve any purpose other than making a person feel bad, which they may already be feeling. Staying connected and in the relationship is key to assessing how things have gone wrong and supporting the staff involved.

Both compassionate and person-centred leadership are research-informed, and I question why both approaches are not more widely used in the NHS. I appreciate that there is an emphasis on targets, performance, and evidence-based practice. I wonder how much this moves us away from the creative, intuitive, and relational approach where attention is paid to discussing how best to work with and for women. Understanding the organisation and the systems in it are relevant to leadership, but not to the cost of the relationships with maternity service users and their primary resource, the staff. The role of a good leader is to model attitudes and behaviour to the people in the organisation.

I think the poignant lyrics of the band Everything but the Girl 'the heart remains a child', are relevant. They can remind us that although the heart can be mature, we rarely act 'grown up' 100 percent of the time, particularly when we feel vulnerable or hurt. It is crucial to notice when we feel small and regress into our younger selves. These are times when we can be guided by wise elders: in other words, those with more experience and wisdom than ourselves. For example, a leader, supervisor, coach, or mentor might offer guidance when we need support and elevation back into our adult selves. When considering examples of wise elders and experienced leaders, people such as Nelson Mandela, Maya Angelou, Brené Brown, and Ken Robinson spring to mind. These leaders have inspired many in their words of wisdom and have therefore been honoured, but not necessarily fully integrated into our approaches to leadership. Perhaps this is a reminder of how difficult it is to practise the discipline of being relational.

4

SPEAKING OUR TRUTHS

'Lightning makes no sound until it strikes.'
Martin Luther King Jr

When all that is left are feelings and memories, where do we go to tell our stories, our truth as we know it? Many people contacted me when I requested experiences from maternity staff of times when they felt supported, inspired, and shown kindness, at work (or not) by colleagues and leaders. Below are the experiences many staff have courageously shared with me.

Jess, midwife

I was having another terrible shift, and had escaped to the toilets for refuge. There, I hunkered down in the cubicle and sobbed. It was only my second week in the job. Out of nowhere I looked up and standing outside, her gentle voice washed over me, enquiring if I was okay. Whenever I felt I was wobbling at work, she always seemed to be there, with an aura of calm. Remembering her words, her kindness, her smile even now years later brings me comfort. She went on to become head of midwifery, and everyone who came into contact with her shared the same story. She listened, made you feel you were worth something, and she made the best cups of tea! That's the kind of leader I want to become.

Anonymous

When I first qualified as a midwife I had high expectations. I was determined that I was only going to give the best care. I was going to be attentive and listen to the needs of each individual family that I came into contact with. It's in my nature to be kind anyway, so it only made sense that that was the kind of midwife I wanted to be. During the first year of being qualified I struggled with this somewhat. Not because I wasn't being kind but because frankly I was struggling to find the time. The workload was so high that it simply didn't leave time for listening. I felt awful, it felt like I was failing every family I came into contact with. I figured that it was because I was a bad midwife, that my time management was poor or because I was so junior, but I remained hopeful that as I became more experienced I would be able manage these things better and I'd finally be able to be the midwife I wanted to be.

Over time things did improve slightly. I became better at managing my time, I became more confident in all of my clinical skills and I actually began to be able to talk to families more about the choices that lay in front of them. I still didn't feel good and I knew that I still wasn't being the midwife I wanted to be, but at least things had improved. However, now there was a new problem. Now that I was able to have more in-depth conversations with families I found that a lot of the time they would want to make choices that weren't within the normal care pathway. I thought this was great at first. It meant that the families I was looking after were finally able to make the choices they truly wanted, it meant that I was finally giving true informed choice, but it soon began to become a problem.

If I was working on the Labour Ward I would inform the midwife in charge and the obstetrician of the decision that had been made, and soon after one of them would come into the room and undo all of my hard work. They would begin to coerce the family into making a choice that better fit with the usual care pathway. It was heartbreaking. I knew it wasn't what they really wanted but I felt powerless to stop it. I couldn't argue with my colleagues because that would have meant the family lost their confidence in the people that were looking after them. Plus, I had to maintain a good working relationship and I didn't want to be seen as a troublemaker.

If I was working on the Birthing Unit, things were slightly different. The midwife in charge would rarely interfere by going in and speaking to the family, but instead I would be pressured into changing their minds. I would be told things like 'You're going to lose your registration if anything happens'. Or 'What's wrong with her? Doesn't she care about her baby?' Every time it happened I would have this sinking feeling in my stomach. I'd be made to feel like a fool for supporting the decision. My confidence was sinking fast.

Going into work became harder and harder. I would have to make a choice each shift – a choice between being accepted by my colleagues or providing good midwifery care. Of course, I always simply wanted to be a good midwife, but I was also a human being. I wanted to feel part of the team. I wanted to feel normal. Plus, these midwives were good people deep down. I started to think that maybe they were right. Maybe I was wrong for supporting families in the way that I was. I became confused and withdrawn. Until one day I found myself becoming like the other midwives. A mother wanted to stay in hospital: she was in early labour but she had had a difficult pregnancy and was very vulnerable. I knew that the right thing was to let her stay, but despite pleading with several of my senior colleagues, they refused. They gave all the usual excuses and I listened. I went back to see this mother and told her she had to leave. As those words left my mouth, I knew that that was it. I simply couldn't do it anymore. I couldn't keep living in this constant state of conflict. So I left.

In the months that followed I went through some dark times. I think I was suffering from burnout and it was only when I began to feel better that I was able to see how bad things had been. My mental health had suffered badly while I was working but I simply hadn't been able to see it at the time. Now, with the benefit of hindsight, I know why. It was because those that were working around me were all going through the same thing. They all felt the same way as me. None of them became midwives with the intention of causing harm or providing bad care. They were simply left with no choice. In the end, they either had to leave or simply give up caring. Continuing to care was what took its toll on me. That inner conflict is something that can only be borne for a certain amount of time before it chips away at you. One day I hope things change but I know that we can't simply tell midwives to 'give better care'. We need to heal these midwives first, we need to show them the nurturing and kindness, so that they can once again be the midwives they've always wanted to be.

Amity Reed, author of *Overdue*

Early in my career, I overheard a midwife describe a vulnerable mother on the postnatal ward who had recently experienced domestic violence by her partner as a 'piece of work' because she was ringing the call bell frequently. She then added, 'If I was her husband, I'd probably have given her a slap too.' Later the same week, I assisted at a forceps birth in which the doctor told the mother I was caring for to 'shut your mouth and push' when she tried to ask a question and did not gain consent before performing an unnecessarily rough vaginal examination. I was so shocked and saddened by what I'd heard in both instances that I was unable to respond. Instead, I walked away with tears in my eyes, wondering how in the world my colleagues, who I knew to be otherwise competent and caring, could say something so awful.

Witnessing these acts of cruelty, alongside the traumatic births, coercion and violations of dignity that were occurring with greater frequency, troubled me greatly. I felt complicit in an abusive system that seemed determined to chew mothers up and spit them out. Increasingly, I saw that it was doing the same to midwives too. A sense of deep sadness, anger, frustration and helplessness began to build in me like layers of sediment, making everything hazy and difficult to navigate. Every time I saw a mother ignored, treated poorly or made to feel small, I felt I'd been kicked in the gut. Every time I saw our inhumane working conditions normalised, or a kind-hearted, outspoken colleague endure relentless bullying, a small piece of my bright, beating heart was chipped away and replaced by something flat and dark. It seemed that trauma was all around me, and now included my own.

Much of what I'd learned at university and from my employer and union over the years about managing stress and trauma in midwifery was about building resilience and practising self-care. Reminders to go for walks, talk to a friend or colleague, practise yoga or meditation and enjoy some downtime to decompress were all around me. I internalised these messages to the point where I felt responsible for my own ability to adapt to and accept the system I worked in. As a result, any lingering negative feelings or experiences felt like a personal failing, not a systemic one. When I took a leave of absence due to work-related stress, anxiety and depression, I was initially embarrassed and ashamed. I was convinced that most of my colleagues would be judging me and deem me weak, wondering why on earth I hadn't learned to keep calm and carry on like the rest of them. Little did I know that many of them were feeling the same as I was, or how many had been off work or left the profession for similar reasons.

The number of messages I received over the course of the next few months and continue to receive today, nearly two years after I left the NHS, still astounds and humbles me. Colleagues I worked with closely and midwives I've never met have all shared their joy and their pain with me, so similar to my own. I read and hear their stories and hold them in my heart, so grateful to be entrusted with their words. We are a silent sisterhood of women grieving damage to or loss of our vocation, hopes, aspirations and dreams. We are a reminder of how vital our services are to society, of how deep the bonds are between midwives and mothers, and why it's so important to *all* of us that we get it right. By sharing our experiences and raising our voices, we raise awareness. Every time we tell our stories, we write a new chapter. Our stories are the key. Our stories are our power.

Jenny Clarke, midwife

I retired from clinical midwifery in the NHS in 2018 because I was bullied. This experience was extremely tough, but two and a half years later I am able to recognise why others chose to target me, and also that this has actually helped me to support others who are going through a difficult time in their own workplace.

Staff trauma stems from repeated exposure to tragic situations, low morale, missed opportunities for counselling, stress, burnout, staff shortages, being bullied and/or undermined, pressure to conform, poor shift patterns, a lack of consideration for work-life balance and many other factors which continue to surface.

Inherent to any organisation's success or failure as an employer is the way it makes its employees feel while they are working there. As some organisations become larger (and/or try to raise their profile) more problems may start to arise, a general air of complacency can follow whereby the people who keep the organisation on its feet may sadly melt into the background. The public face of the organisation may seem rather perfect, but behind the scenes cracks appear because staff are not being cared for. Incidents become more commonplace and a culture of blame transpires. While the public view of the organisation may seem positive, the reality is that staff are unhappy.

If we think of a happy place where we feel safe and nurtured many of us will think of our own homes or simply being alongside someone who cares for us and this is how a maternity service should feel – safe, nurturing, open and welcome yet a place to hide away from the hustle and bustle. A place where we are allowed to be our own individual selves that rejoice in our diversity.

When women are looking at which maternity unit to choose, a good question to ask would be 'How do you care for your midwives, maternity support workers, cleaners, clerical staff and obstetricians?' because when employees are nurtured in the work environment, they are more likely to give good care. An organisation that prides itself on giving good care to its staff will transmit a positive vibe and a warm welcome, for both staff and women.

KM, anaesthetist

I love my job and at times the connection it allows me to create with patients. Sitting with them and listening to their worries about their birth, and working together to try and help them feel calmer and more in control. I had spent quite a while with a mum and her partner. Both had been traumatised by their previous birth, and understandably were anxious not to repeat it. We had a plan, they were happy, and I really wanted to make this experience as healing as it could be for them.

We were all prepped and the section began. Everything looked good, mum and partner were happy. Then the obstetrician openly began to criticise the midwife who we all worked with. One of the midwives attempted to change the subject, but he persisted, more vehemently than before! He started to attack her personally. I can only describe it as the feeling in the room changed, it suddenly felt very tense. Everyone was silent. It was like none of us knew what to do. He had centre stage. I looked down at the parents and we started to talk, I was trying to distract them from him. The cry of their baby broke the tension.

I visited them on the ward shortly after. They shared how they had absorbed the tension in the operating theatre. Although they hadn't been traumatised by the experience, they were disappointed by it, and angry that 'this doctor couldn't control himself'. They both were relieved to have had their baby delivered, and had felt fearful to say anything. I walked away from them feeling like not only had I let them down, gone back on my promise to make the birth as healing as it could have been, I also had not stood up for my colleague, defended her. I wish I could say that I learned that day to stick up for those I work with, but I can't. I don't know what to say or how to say it. I've become a bystander of bullying acts and I feel deeply ashamed about that.

Beatrice Bennett, student midwife

At the university where I study, continuity of carer through caseholding is promoted to students through the three years of the midwifery course. In my first year, I provided continuity to a woman who was expecting her fifth child. Providing continuity to this woman encouraged the development of a close trusting relationship between the two of us. Just a few months into my midwifery training, this woman in my casehold was admitted to the maternity unit with severe abdominal pain while I was on shift. The woman was very unwell, experiencing a placental abruption and sadly, as a result an intrauterine foetal death. Watching the woman go through such a traumatic experience, including finding out her baby had died and being on the intensive care unit, has stayed with me throughout my training. At the time, I had such little knowledge about the unfolding situation I struggled to understand what was happening. I worked overtime to be with her to make sure she was not alone, mentally and physically exhausting myself. I had so many unanswered questions, including questioning my ability to cope with such events and my ability to ever be a midwife. The situation shook me so much and I was so full of doubt. I left the maternity unit that day a completely different version of myself and wondering if I would ever go back.

On returning home, I contacted my personal tutor at the university to let her know what had happened and to make a decision about when and if I would return to practice. I went to meet her, ready to share my doubts about my capability and if I was pursuing the right career. The way she spoke to me that day completely changed my perspective. We did not learn about complications of bereavement care until our second year, but she took the opportunity to teach me everything I needed to know to understand the situation I had been in and shared with me a similar experience she had been in. She gave me the time and space I needed to debrief and reflect on the situation and helped create a supportive plan for me to return to practice after a few days away. As a result of her support, I felt able to return to my placement to visit the woman I had been caring for and support her in the bereavement suite. I also felt empowered to advocate for the woman to ensure the care she received was centred around her needs and wishes. She expressed how grateful she was to me for coming to support her. I was so proud of the care I had been able to provide, considering a week earlier I had questioned if I was capable of doing this job. This year, I was fortunate enough to support the same woman in her next pregnancy and birth.

What I felt would be the end of my career actually became the most pivotal experience for me in my whole three years of training. A few months into my training, I had found my voice as an advocate for women. I developed the strength to put my own feelings aside to provide the best care I can for families, but to not ignore those thoughts after work and compromise my own mental wellbeing. My personal tutor warned me against the word resilience as she feared that we are expected to be able to cope without regard for our feelings, reminding me that we should be upset when things go wrong because we are supposed to care about the women we care for. However, we do need to be able to process and manage these thoughts to be able to carry on caring for women and their families in their times of need. The support I received from my personal tutor and my colleagues allowed me to continue with my training and ensured that in future situations, my ability to care for women and balance my own mental wellbeing has not been compromised. Without being surrounded by supportive colleagues and university staff, I believe I would be in a very different situation now.

Sorry – a story by Alice Bell, GP and runner-up in the BMA's 2020 writing competition

She stood just outside the room, blocking my exit so when I opened the door, hoping to have a moment to process what had happened, I almost walked into her.

My damp scrubs stuck to the small of my back. My legs ached. My hands still smarted from the hot water that had washed off the dried blood which had speckled my forearms and trickled inside my gloves to my fingernails. Fatigue and hunger were making me feel nauseous. A buzzer sounded up the corridor.

A man walked past, carrying a large silver balloon with a small bear with 'Congratulations' on it. I moved aside to let him into the room I had just left.

She was tall, her dark hair drawn back, and lips pursed. Almost graceful. Her left hand rested on her left hip through her blue scrubs, whilst with her right hand she formed a wagging finger at my eye level.

Her blue eyes looked directly into mine.

'Naughty. Tut tut. That was entirely your fault,' she said. The fluorescent bulbs glared and reflected off the linoleum floor.

The senior midwife stood next to her looking on.

'Sorry' I reflexively said, feeling my eyes pricking.

I turned to the midwife.

'Sarah, please let theatre know we've got a case. Possible third degree tear'.

Then I had no option but to accompany her to the handover room.

'I don't know what you were thinking pulling down for so long, no wonder she tore,' she said.

I sat down behind her on one of the chairs, tucking my legs under the desk whilst feeling my lower back sag into the chair. My mouth was dry. I can't remember what I said in response. Perhaps I said nothing.

I remember the feeling as if it was yesterday, ashamed, guilty, exposed. I was ill-equipped to deal with it.

I couldn't formulate a response.

Feeling numb, I went back into the room to explain what had happened to the mother. The balloon bobbed cheerfully at the head of the bed. The room was warm but her new clean white sheets felt cool as I placed a hand on the bed to keep me steady.

I could see a pile of bloodied sheets in the corner of the room. The used metal instruments clinked noisily as they were tipped into the bin. The placenta made a wet slapping sound as it was placed in the shining stainless steel kidney dish before being taken to the sluice. Her baby was calm, snuffling and sucking its hand.

I can't remember her name and barely remember her face. I do remember her bewildered look, the exhausted euphoria that comes with having a new baby. The distracted acceptance of the events as I explained them: that when I helped her deliver her baby, she had torn. She signed the consent form.

I didn't apologise.

I didn't apologise.

A short time later in theatre, I assisted in repairing the tear. I watched as she meticulously brought tissues together to close the mother's wound. I helped to hold this suture here and cut that suture there. I helped mop up blood when it obscured a clear view of the skin. I wiped the blood away afterwards and counted the swabs with the scrub nurse. I gave the notes to her so she could write up the work she had done.

Later that day, as I was cycling home through the Saturday morning traffic and remnants of others' revelry the night before, I would think about her comment as we walked away from theatres; patting me on the back, she sarcastically told me not to make the same mistake again because she didn't want to have to clear up my mess again the coming night. Again, I apologised.

I often think about that night shift. It felt seismic in its effect. I think about that mother, who was owed the apology. I think about the apology I gave away so cheaply to someone who didn't deserve it. And, finally, I think about why I decided to leave obstetrics.

Reflection on my story 'Sorry'

When I wrote this piece, I was in the weeks after delivery of my second child, which was not a traumatic event. I was responding to a writing competition with the title 'Sorry', and before I knew what I was writing, this story came to the forefront of my mind. Thinking back on it now, I feel mostly anger and frustration that I did not stand up for myself, or apologise to the patient, or approach a mentor to discuss what had happened. The feeling of shame and guilt after this event is something that can still feel very real, and I am sure that this was a significant contributory factor to me leaving obstetrics.

I have been surprised by the reaction to this piece. I have been contacted by many previous obstetric colleagues who have expressed their sympathy but also anger that this situation happened; these same colleagues have told me that they have experienced similar behaviour from others at work.

Dr Sally Pezaro, midwife and academic

I dreamt of becoming a midwife ever since my brother was born when I was aged just four. Utterly fascinated, I watched in awe as he grew and then emerged into the world. I read my mother's baby books cover to cover. My dream of becoming a midwife came true during my mid-twenties. I had never felt so full of wonder and promise before. I was determined to change the world. Over the next few years, my enthusiasm wore down. I experienced one negative comment and/or behaviour after another. This was not what I had dreamt of after all. I felt disempowered and unable to speak up. Excitement and anticipation became replaced with anxiety and dread.

Following a serious and traumatic clinical incident at work I then quickly became very ill. It was the darkest time in my life as my symptomatic behaviours caused me to lose my fitness to practise. I was subsequently diagnosed with two separate mental health conditions. In partnership with the Nursing and Midwifery Council (NMC) I then worked hard to regain my health and thus my fitness to practise. I was consequently able to return to the profession I love. I now frequently draw upon the insights gained from these experiences as a fitness to practise panellist on the NMC's investigating committee, in my research and in my teaching. I am now dedicated to securing the wellbeing of midwives, as this will be integral to the flourishment of the profession and the safety and quality of midwifery services overall. I began this journey by securing a PhD scholarship at Coventry University.

Dr Ruth-Anna, obstetrician

Sitting at home on my sofa under a duvet, I felt absolutely lousy as my two small kids played noisily around me. I wasn't totally sure why I felt so ill – some of it was undoubtedly down to being seven weeks pregnant. But I felt shivery and shaky as well as the nausea and exhaustion I knew well from my previous pregnancies. Just the previous day I'd had an email from work saying I had been exposed to confirmed flu A and they recommended I take Tamiflu. So maybe it was the flu. But it was a bank holiday, and I was due in to work a night shift in just a few hours' time. As every doctor knows, calling in sick at the last minute for bank holiday nights creates a huge problem, as your colleagues and seniors scrabble around for locum cover which often can't be found. I messaged around my colleagues, to see if anyone could cover the shift, but they were all busy, or out of town with family. So I swallowed some paracetamol and dragged myself in to work.

Three weeks later, I rushed into antenatal clinic, having dropped my older two children at school breakfast club and raced to get to the hospital on time. My first patient was still with the healthcare assistant having her blood pressure checked so I took a couple of minutes to look up the investigations for the baby we had cared for that Easter night, who had been playing on my mind. Reading through his MRI report, I felt as if I'd been winded. Up until then I'd managed to convince myself that this baby was going to be like so many others we encounter in obstetrics – delivered very unwell but miraculously with little or no ongoing damage. Not this time. Tears flowed as I sat on my own, my fingers shaking as I texted one of my friends with the news that a baby would have severe brain damage as a result of my actions, or rather, as a result of my inaction that night.

I have never wanted more strongly to be able to turn back time. I stumbled through the rest of the clinic, unable to articulate my distress to the consultant or SHO I was working alongside. Hours became days. The baby and his family occupied pretty much my every waking thought, eating into time at home with my own children, who I struggled to enjoy, feeling guilty for their health and happiness. I struggled not to blame the new baby I was growing myself for the string of events. After all, if I hadn't been in the early weeks of my own pregnancy, and feeling horribly unwell, and on nights, maybe I would have made better decisions and acted faster? Time and time again I went over my choices and decision-making that night. I reviewed the CTGs so many times that I could almost draw every line by heart.

I wandered around in a fog at work, going through the motions, but struggled with any kind of decision-making process. An astute consultant who knew me well noticed this and suggested a few days off work. Initially I resisted, terrified that at home I would just dwell on things even more and fall off a cliff edge into an abyss, but a week of walks, reading, sleeping and seeing friends did help me start to move on from constantly thinking about that night and its long-term implications.

About a month down the line, still struggling to sleep, eat properly or focus on much else, I referred myself to the Professional Support Unit at London Deanery, who recommended I self-refer to the Practitioner Health Programme service for doctors struggling with stress, depression or other mental health problems. These both provided a vital support and, along with my family and friends, kept me in work and with my head just about above water. However, the feeling of guilt was all pervasive; that I deserved to feel awful, that any distress was of my own making; that it was nothing in comparison to what the family were going through; that I didn't deserve to be helped in any way.

Every time I started to get back to any kind of 'normal', I had to metaphorically rip the plaster back off – to write my statement, to attend a 'serious incident' review and round table meeting, to read the resulting report several months later and discuss it with my supervisor, to discuss it at my annual appraisal, and, two days before starting my own maternity leave, to meet the family and their baby face to face – which was absolutely one of the hardest things I've ever done. I was given the choice to stay away, but turned it down, as I felt I owed the family any answers I could possibly provide. In retrospect, I think I forced myself to go as a kind of punishment. And punishing it was, though nothing I felt I didn't deserve.

The first time I looked after a patient in similar circumstances I felt utter panic rising in my throat. I looked for the first excuse to deliver the baby as soon as possible and finally understood the perspective of being that person that everyone else thinks is over-reacting. I pore over CTGs a lot more now. I get second opinions on things I never would have considered doing. I definitely practise more defensively. Although my mental wellbeing is much better, it's something I still think about frequently and it can still intrude into my thoughts unprovoked.

In retrospect I can see that what happened that night fitted the multi-factorial Swiss Cheese model of error causation to a T. There are many pieces of the jigsaw that I can now see contributed to the outcome. Rationally with time this has helped me process things although the guilt is still very strong.

It's 12 years since my first job in obstetrics and yet until a few years ago I'd never heard the term 'second victim'. We all know the statistics about medical errors, yet as doctors we rarely discuss them in anything other than the most abstract terms. These are things that happen to 'other people' – and, we assume, probably to incompetent, lazy or uncaring doctors. When I experienced it myself, some other colleagues finally started telling me their own stories. Hearing other doctors who I hugely respect talking honestly about their mistakes was one of the most important contributors to me still being in the speciality and able to see a future for myself in obstetrics. It's absolutely not easy. Egos are fragile, medicine is famously hierarchical and in many ways it functions due to a belief that doctors, especially senior doctors, are infallible. This erroneous belief not only damages individuals, who feel they are alone in their distress, but is also a huge factor in missed institutional learning.

It is over four years now since this little boy was born. I can't turn back time, but I can throw myself into doing everything I can within my power to reduce the number of other families who are affected. This is my promise to him, and to his family.

I have tried to channel my guilt and sadness into positive improvements in the care I offer to patients and to my colleagues. I have become absolutely passionate about trying to change the culture of presenteeism among medical staff and encouraging colleagues to call in sick if they are unwell. I've developed a strong interest in human factors – the real, human variables that are present in almost every single adverse medical outcome, and I am now studying for an MSc in Patient Safety and Clinical Human Factors alongside finishing my training. I have spent 15 months working at the Healthcare Safety Investigation Branch, developing my knowledge and skills in human factors focused investigations. I passionately believe that doctors and midwives do not go to work aiming to cause harm. As a profession we have a long way to go to improve awareness and training around human factors and how to mitigate for them.

I have somehow managed to hold on to my love of acute, high-risk obstetrics. Many colleagues, both doctors and midwives, have not been so fortunate. Careers, and even lives, are ended due to both adverse outcomes, and the way they are then handled. It makes me wonder why we wait for tragedy to strike to acknowledge our own fallibility and humanity.

Recently, it does feel like the tide is turning. Human factors are finally making it into medical curricula. Hospitals are starting to appreciate the need to look at systemic level changes in their incident reviews. We owe it to our colleagues, as well as our patients, to keep this momentum going.

Hannah Horne, Deputy Head of Midwifery

I will never forget the day I answered my phone to a colleague who was distraught – she, through sobs, explained how her best friend was threatening to commit suicide – she begged me to help. Her best friend was a fellow midwife who had been involved in a serious incident which had a catastrophic outcome.

As a senior manager within an NHS Trust that was under significant scrutiny, I was becoming used to dealing with complex and unpredictable situations, but this phone call scared me. I promised to help even though I wasn't sure where to start! I desperately called occupational health and human resources for help and their only suggestion was to call an ambulance to attend her!

Despite the advice to call an ambulance I knew that I had to make contact with this midwife. With a shaky hand and a racing heart I picked up the phone and called her. We knew each other but mainly as distant acquaintances – I was a manager and she was a Band 6 midwife. We hadn't worked together but had seen each other at work and were always pleasant. I explained that I had been contacted by her friend and that she was worried. To my surprise the midwife thanked me for calling and began to share her feelings and thoughts with me... I just listened. I listened with tears running down my face as she described how she was feeling, how she deserved to feel this way because she was involved in an incident. I didn't interrupt, I just let her talk – there were moments that she was quiet and during these moments I explained that what she said was confidential and safe.

These words gave her the permission to explore her feelings. The midwife felt lost both at work and at home, she couldn't make sense of what had happened and her involvement in the incident. She had discussed with her doctor who suggested that she take some time off work sick. The midwife didn't want to do this – she felt that being at home alone made her worse.

When the midwife finished talking I validated that I had heard what she was really saying – she thanked me through sobs as she realised that she had finally been heard despite speaking to a number of friends. I asked her to come and work with me. I explained that although we can't take back what happened during the incident we could change things for the future. She was really excited about the opportunities that I was offering and jumped at the chance to work with me. We took each day as it came and focused on small projects.

Over time the midwife grew from a scared, shy and timid woman to a strong, empowered and focused individual. I regularly text her to say how proud I am of her... she turned her negative experience into something positive. She has written a number of guidelines, completed audits and has taught fellow midwives about her journey. Thanks to her we have made many significant and sustainable changes within our Trust – all that she needed was for someone to listen and really hear her!

I recently received this text from her:

'Before you listened to me I felt lost, I was contemplating giving up midwifery and taking early retirement! I felt like I didn't deserve to be a midwife. But now I have never been so happy and fulfilled in my job. I am going to apply for a promotion – I have so much to give. Thank you!'

Nicole Rajan-Brown, second-year student midwife

As midwives, we live in a constant battle between professional and organisational values. I have felt this strongly as a student midwife, also being bound to the expectations of mentors and universities. There is a constant feeling of wanting to remain true to the reasons I entered into the profession, maintaining true midwifery, while avoiding institutionalisation.

I have experienced midwives and doctors carrying out

membrane sweeps as an extension of a vaginal examination without consent, the use of derogatory, outdated terminology, inaccurate information being provided, and coercive control. These experiences have led to me questioning practice, and my role in these events.

There are many barriers to speaking up as a student: hierarchy, bullying, the culture of normalising these events. Bullying between qualified professionals and students is not always overt, often it is in the form of microaggressions, undermining confidence. Furthermore, there is a fear that speaking will impact on training; those with whom these conversations could be had, or those whose practice you would question, are the same people supporting and signing off the achievement of your competencies. Without keeping your head down, there is a risk of not successfully completing placements, or making them more difficult experiences. All these factors contribute to feeling unable express concerns. This has left me often feeling uncomfortable, with feelings of guilt and complicity to poor care, feeling I am letting families down by not speaking out when I know quality, respectful care is not being provided.

I have been fortunate to encounter midwives who are role models for the type of midwife I aspire to become; midwives who encourage, empower and respect. These midwives have advised me to reflect on practice witnessed as a student, considering which good practices to assume, and which poor practices to vehemently and consciously avoid. That it is important to focus on building trust with mentors, so that a level of independence is obtained, to provide woman-centred, truly midwifery-based care. I have found this has allowed me to support active positions on labour ward during continuous monitoring, and provide the latest evidence-based information to give true informed consent, taking these moments to practise the midwifery skills I wish to develop.

Although I could somewhat accept this reflective pathway towards the beginning of my training, as I progress through my training this is no longer sufficient. Waiting until qualification is not enough. In addition to the fear, when frequently working with different mentors, inaccessibility of trusted individuals, and local Trust politics, support can be hard to access. Although this reflection and desire to improve my own practice is positive for my development as a midwife, the pressure inevitably has had some mental strain, often unable to shake certain experiences from my mind, wondering how I could have acted differently, and the consequences – good and bad. Promising myself next time I will find my voice.

The student-mother relationship has its challenges; sometimes being 'with women' means taking a step back, putting the mother's needs over my need for experience. Other times, this means putting my head above the parapet, putting my own discomfort and potential personal consequences aside to put the woman's needs first. The former can be done with relative ease, the latter is something I battle with each shift.

With the growth of social media, connecting with midwives, student and qualified, is made easier, garnering support locally, nationally and internationally. Finding my tribe, those from whom I can gain support and advice, is increasingly easily accessible. I hope to learn from these professionals and, with their support, find my voice to speak out, and remain true to the midwifery skills I so desire to develop.

5

THE TIDE OF CHANGE

'And in your darkest moments,
When it feels like no one could possibly understand
The storm you're weathering,
Turn to words – to music, to poetry,
To books, to quotes, to conversations.
As you read, as you listen, as you speak,
The words will remind you
That someone else does, in fact, understand;
That you're, in fact, never alone in this storm;
And that, just like every other season,
This too shall pass.'

Leslie Dwight

Things were tough for many staff working in maternity before Covid-19 hit. During the pandemic I heard a range of experiences from staff: some colleagues, teams, and organisations pulled together in acts of solidarity, and some (for the first time) felt supported and valued. Others, however, felt more isolated, alone, frightened, and consequently, their mental wellbeing suffered. A positive outcome from the pandemic is growing awareness, discussions, and plans reflecting the importance of establishing and maintaining a psychologically healthy workforce in the NHS. However, to achieve this we must consider several factors.

System-level changes
Changing the culture

Most maternity staff enter a culture they have inherited and weren't necessarily part of creating that culture. However, being part of the system means that you are now part of the culture, and there are things we can all do to change it. Although creating a positive working culture starts with leaders, you don't need to be in a leadership position to contribute. This can be done in the hundreds of daily interactions you have with colleagues. Most organisations have many subcultures, and the power of these can force positive changes, or, conversely, sabotage quality improvements.

There are many aspects of maternity services that are great and work well. So, it isn't necessarily the case that radically overhauling the whole culture is needed, rather considering what needs to change and what can be implemented to ensure the change is maintained.

Working in maternity can be physically and emotionally demanding. This is partly because staff support women and families who might be experiencing emotional distress or who have had previous psychological trauma. One way for an organisation to facilitate staff to support these families empathetically and compassionately, without experiencing burnout, vicarious trauma, or emotional stress, is to prioritise staff wellbeing proactively.

This can be achieved by creating a culture that accepts the challenges of working in maternity services, and expects that care will not go as planned sometimes. That staff will require a level of emotional support throughout their career. Also, supporting mental wellbeing should be rewarded, not seen as a weakness or used as a weapon to belittle colleagues. In the absence of such a culture, staff must rely on their own methods to cope with getting through a shift or manage how they feel when they return home, meaning they are often left with difficult thoughts and feelings. The organisation doesn't emotionally equip them to work in a highly challenging system throughout their training and subsequent career. Instead, they are left to go like lambs to the slaughter.

Emily, a newly qualified midwife, begins her new job. One month into her post, she has learned that she is 'with paperwork', not 'with woman'. Her role is learning to juggle endless tasks, prioritising those most in need, getting used to not going to the toilet much, having little to eat or drink for 12 hours, and coming home with her feet, back, and muscles burning with tiredness. Choosing between caring wholeheartedly for women or completing administrative jobs is a regular dilemma each shift. Maybe it will get better with experience and time.

Fast-forward one year. Emily now feels like she is constantly exhausted. She feels she has little emotional energy left to give to her partner, family, or friends. Emily is increasingly overwhelmed, and a few months into her new role, she had started to have a couple of glasses of wine after each shift to 'wind down'. She now has a bottle of wine after each day and night shift finishes. Emily is worried about how much she is drinking, how she has come to hide it from her partner, and the guilt and shame she is feeling about it, but what's the alternative? She feels like she has nowhere to turn.

Take a moment and consider this: what if Emily was your sister, daughter, mum, colleague, friend, or partner, and she shared this. How would you respond? Most people would probably respond with empathy, compassion, and concern, expecting that Emily would need support. Sadly, in my experience, Emily's story is a familiar one, and too often understanding is not the response from the wider organisation. Dr Sally Pezaro, a registered midwife, NMC panellist, a fellow of the Royal College of Midwives and academic at Coventry University and her colleagues have researched substance misuse within midwifery. Although their findings are not yet published, evidence suggests that midwives with problematic substance use engage in this as a coping mechanism. Burnout can often contribute to problematic substance misuse, and so understanding the prevalence of this within midwifery is vital for staff wellbeing and quality of care. We need to identify ways of ensuring staff can access the support and treatment they need without fear, stigma or judgement from their colleagues or organisation.

When someone contacts me for support, this will have taken immense courage and interpersonal risk. They usually have deliberated, questioned, and doubted whether they should text, email or phone. I use the word courage intentionally, because that is what I witness. They choose to do something different: acknowledging their pain, difficulties, or stress and seeking another way of being. This is not an easy thing to do. The culture in many maternity organisations normalises secrecy, silences staff, and responds with judgement, usually in the form of 'that's the way it is, and you just need to get on with it'. This culture is not conducive to optimising staff mental wellbeing.

Invest in staff

A good example of this is the Camden Coalition of Healthcare Providers in New Jersey,[1] which has implemented innovative practices to enhance staff wellbeing, encouraging them to engage in self-care practices and use mental health support services. They contract an independent company to provide these, and each employee has up to $2,000 to spend annually on their mental wellbeing, in addition to their standard health insurance cover.

The wellbeing culture is embedded in clinicians' workload policies to avoid burnout from long hours and promote a work/life balance. Staff are encouraged to leave their work mobile phones in the office when not at work (administrative staff enforce this by leaving them on charge overnight). The care team staff only see patients within a 40-hour working week, and at times when staff have worked overtime, colleagues cover their workload to ensure the 40-hour working week is maintained.

At the beginning of each day, there is a short morning 'huddle'. These have a different theme and are opportunities for staff to acknowledge something positive a colleague did, physically move, or solve a difficult issue, for example. Also, weekly care planning meetings provide an opportunity to discuss patient care and are another space for staff to support one another and process professional or personal difficulties.

A psychologist has been employed, their role being to support staff and ensure that their mental wellbeing is prioritised. Additionally, staff are taught that they can't care for patients without first caring for themselves, and so the psychologist helps them to establish professional boundaries to prioritise wellness and reduce burnout.

Opportunities are created for staff to spend time together away from their working environment to strengthen relationships. No meetings are held on Fridays for any staff member to encourage them to complete administrative tasks before the weekend.

This organisation financially invests in each employee. The infrastructure, policies, and resources are implemented at each level to ensure that staff wellbeing is being prioritised and a nurturing culture is created.

Just Culture

When teams work in a psychologically safe environment, colleagues can be open and honest with one another. They don't necessarily have higher numbers of medical errors, but they may *report* more because they can talk openly about mistakes and work to find ways to prevent them.

When an incident does occur, having a Just Culture model embedded in the organisation helps individuals feel confident to report when events did not go as expected so that they can be better understood. NHSS Improvement has published 'A Just Culture Guide', which aims to support managers to respond to staff involved in patient safety incidents and to ensure they are treated fairly.

For a Just Culture to be truly embedded in an organisation, managers, senior leaders, and board members need to be fully on board and model the behaviours that the culture promotes. There are some great examples of Just and Learning cultures in organisations in the UK.

Over the past few years, MerseyCare has worked with Professor Sidney Dekker, author of the best-selling book *Just Culture*. They initially piloted a Restorative Just Culture, focusing on healing rather than hurting those involved in adverse events. Rather than begin an HR investigation immediately (which they were doing previously), they prioritised seeing what support was required following the incident and who was best placed to provide it. The number of safety incident reports increased, while disciplinaries and suspensions reduced.[2] This approach is now integral in each part of the organisation, and is supported by, for example, appointing Just Culture ambassadors, helping managers support staff differently, and being aware of the language used to reinforce a focus on learning 'when care doesn't go to plan'.

Shame and blame don't make staff practise more safely. When some part of the care being delivered falls below the standards staff, patients, and the organisation expect, the culture can serve to alleviate the potential emotional burden those involved might take on.

Promoting wellbeing within teams

'It's all about teamwork', 'there's no "I" in team', 'you need to be a team player'. Both subtly and overtly staff are fed the message that being in and positively contributing to a team is the linchpin of healthcare. This is true to an extent. Stressed staff can become impatient and unkind to their colleagues, and these behaviours are contagious. Poor teamwork is the most significant contributor to absenteeism in medical staff, more so than work overload.[3] Therefore, it's essential to pay attention to the quality of colleague relationships and working environment. These can prevent or contribute to levels of stress, burnout, or secondary trauma in colleagues.[4]

Reflective practice groups

It is widely accepted that having a safe space where staff can share the emotional, personal, and ethical challenges of working in healthcare can positively affect their wellbeing, benefitting patients.

Schwartz Rounds were created in the USA, and although there is limited evidence of their efficacy, attendance at them has been associated with many benefits. Some of these include better teamwork, reduced stress in staff, improved compassion for patients, and positively impact on organisational culture.[6,7] Rounds are one intervention that provides a structured forum where all staff, clinical and non-clinical, can regularly discuss the emotional and psychological impact of their work. It is encouraged that staff from a range of positions attend, and there is no pressure to contribute verbally. Such rounds are already running regularly across 182 Trusts in the NHS.[5] Some teams meet monthly or bi-monthly. In this reflective space, staff listen to colleagues sharing the challenges they face at work, which can help normalise some of the emotions involved when working in a demanding environment.

One size doesn't fit all. So rounds should be used in conjunction with other staff wellbeing interventions and organisational initiatives to address environmental and cultural factors that affect wellbeing.[8]

Clinical supervision

As psychologists, we are encouraged and expected to receive clinical supervision regularly throughout our careers. It is not a method to manage the content of work. Instead, it ensures individuals are practising safely, developing as practitioners, and maintaining their wellbeing.

A change in legislation has meant that since 2017 midwives also receive restorative clinical supervision. As part of the A-EQUIP model, led by professional midwifery advocates (PMA), midwives are offered a safe space to process their experiences and reflect on their practice. It is hoped this will improve their working life and minimise the impact of stress and burnout. However, this relies on a trusting and respectful relationship with the supervisor, whose role is to create a safe and nurturing space where the supervisee feels listened to and valued.

Supervision can increase self-awareness, reflection, and interpersonal skills. It is an opportunity to use the supervisee's present-moment reflections of emotional responses to raise their experiential awareness and lead to learning.[9] This can serve to help staff to connect with how they are feeling, explore why they might be feeling like that, and create ways to manage these feelings. Without focusing on reflective practice, there is a danger that staff use supervision to tell stories: for example, 'a family came onto the labour ward, and this happened...'. Although storytelling is part of supervision, it is essential that the supervisor supports staff to gently 'turn in' to themselves and connect with their own experience of what happened, what this felt like for them, and the meaning they made of this. Some positive markers of stress reduction in midwives are their ability to influence the care they provide and the decisions made at work.[10] Restorative supervision also offers an opportunity to reflect on why they have performed as they have and factors that might have influenced those decisions.

Understandably, for many people new to supervision, it can feel foreign to sit with another and explore the impact of work-related experiences. So, one way to think of it is getting to know yourself better, so you can offer the best care to those you support. However, this requires the organisation to expect this from staff, and that the organisational culture positively promotes it. Get creative: if sitting face to face feels too intense, try walking together.

Debriefing

When care doesn't go as expected, staff are often offered a debrief session. Its purpose is not to recycle the events that happened. Rather it is an opportunity to mitigate the potential psychological impact on staff. It is peer-driven and should be led by a therapist, psychologist, or trained maternity worker. For some, healing begins in a moment of connection with another, found in crisis, which debriefing can facilitate. However, there is no conclusive evidence that psychological debriefing after an incident is effective and it can worsen the distress of those involved.[11]

Rather than having one-off resources or support, thinking about how a support culture is embedded into an organisation will undoubtedly be advantageous when staff need it the most. One approach won't suit every person, and everyone will respond differently following a difficult event. Having a range of supportive options that staff can access is more likely to be beneficial to support their general mental wellbeing.

Individual approaches

Some staff understandably feel eroded by their organisation's practices and the unhelpful teachings they have encountered from others. Nonetheless, we all have the power to change our practices, engender self-compassion and manage challenging emotions that might compromise our mental wellbeing.

Meet your basic needs: HALT

It sounds simple, doesn't it! Make sure you eat well, stay hydrated, and take a break while at work.

When I first started supporting maternity staff, I vividly recall an experienced midwife sharing her experience of working a 13-hour shift. She told me that she had only eaten a Mars bar, hadn't had anything to drink, and felt utterly humiliated when halfway through her shift she didn't make it to the toilet in time and urinated in her scrubs. I couldn't believe what I was hearing, but over the years, sadly, I have heard similar stories about the basic needs of staff not being met.

Those working in safety-related industries are familiar with the acronym HALT (hungry, angry, late, tired), and know that when one or more of these factors is present, individuals are more likely to make mistakes. These industries therefore have systems in place to safeguard against the impact of HALT. Many maternity staff are feeling the strain of not having proper breaks and meals (hungry), feeling angry about not being able to provide the care they want to (angry), are under constant time pressures (late), and are tired at the end of their shift if not before (tired). Here are some suggestions that might help look after your mind and body before and after a shift.

Before and during a shift[12]

- Eat a meal that releases energy slowly, like wholegrain foods.
- Pack snacks that are accessible, like fruit, snack bars, chopped vegetables, unsalted nuts.
- Bring a meal with you to work that is high in protein to calm cravings, particularly if you're working a night shift.
- Avoid lots of caffeine – fatigue is a common withdrawal symptom.
- Drink plenty of water.
- If possible, having a 15–20 minute nap during your night shift can improve alertness.

- If you're going to sleep after your shift has ended, try to eat 1–2 hours before that time.

After a shift

- Do you feel able to drive home safely?
- Engage in an activity that helps you unwind and destress. This could be having a bath, walking, listening to some music or a podcast, or doing some gentle yoga.
- Avoid drinking alcohol or taking substances.
- If possible, try to make the room you're relaxing and sleeping in as dark as possible.
- Tempting as it might be, try not to take your phone to bed.
- If you get into bed and your mind is racing, don't lie there tossing and turning. If you're not asleep after 20–30 minutes, get up and do something relaxing until you feel tired enough to try and sleep. If you awaken and are struggling to get back to sleep, this also applies.

There is a groundswell of support for staff taking their breaks, with campaigns starting like #giveusabreak.[13] I think this is an important part of changing the culture within healthcare: it needs to be expected that staff will have their breaks, and systems need to be in place to support this. For example, at the beginning of each shift, someone should be allocated to ensure everyone on the team has their break. It could even be part of the organisation's strategy to ensure that patient safety is maintained. Many colleagues will employ a range of methods to ensure they eat well, are hydrated, relax after their shift, and sleep. This is another opportunity for shared learning: colleagues can get to know what others do to look after themselves before, during, and after their shifts.

LOVE

Dare I use the 'L' word? Let me explain a little more. For over 15 years, I have been practising Acceptance and Commitment Therapy (said as 'ACT', all one word). In a nutshell, clients are taught to accept their internal experiences (emotions, thinking, memories, and bodily sensations) and commit to behaving in a way that is in line with what is important in their lives (values).

For example, imagine having the thought, 'I just can't face another day at work'. This creates feelings of anxiety, anticipating what will unfold on the next shift at work. The person might feel like they want to ring in sick or have a few glasses of wine or other substance to 'numb' the difficult thoughts/feelings. ACT would aim to support the person to accept their thoughts and learn to tolerate the feelings of anxiety, for example by grounding to the present moment (mindfulness), then go into work and behave in a way that's important to them (work-related values), while also being kind and caring to themselves (self-related values). It might sound relatively easy to achieve, but if you're an ACT novice, then like any new skill, it takes lots of practice.

I would invite you to try the following:

- Notice when your thoughts become loud.
- What do they say, and when are they most likely to say it? (Is it when you're tired, feeling stressed, or worried?)
- How do you respond? (Anxious, frightened, sad, frustrated.)
- What might be a different response to practise? (7–11 breathing – see page 99 – mantra, e.g., 'this will pass', or just notice that is what your mind is doing.)

As convincing as our minds can be, thoughts and feelings are not facts. Furthermore, minds can't tell the future. They might say tomorrow's shift will be stressful, or the family in room six will be 'difficult' to manage, but this is not certain. Reminding ourselves of this can be helpful to support having a different relationship with our thoughts and feelings.

Values are like our compass in life. They differ from goals because a goal can be achieved; it can be ticked off the list. What can often anchor individuals in the moment, when their thoughts become loud and hook them in, is to know their values and which behaviours reflect what is important in their personal and working lives. For example, someone's work-related values might be to be patient, caring, and kind. Some behaviours that match the type of maternity worker they want to be could be: to allow colleagues/families to speak without interrupting (patient), to smile, make eye contact, have a gentle tone of voice (caring), and offer a hug/cup of tea to a colleague who looks stressed and reassures an anxious mum (kind). So, when feeling stressed, it's about learning to tolerate this feeling and still behave in a values-based way.

LOVE (Living Our Values Everyday) usually results in individuals feeling happier and more fulfilled in their life. As Steve Hayes, one of the founders of ACT, says, 'love isn't everything, it's the only thing'. I have to say, I wholeheartedly agree.

Moments of calm

In recent years there has been a growing interest in mindfulness interventions. When feeling stressed, most people function on autopilot and can feel caught up in their experience. Mindfulness is *a way of paying attention. It means consciously bringing awareness to our experience, in the present moment, without making judgements about it'.*[14] Regularly practising mindfulness has positively affected a range of cognitive and emotional difficulties, including rumination, worry, and anxiety.[15]

It sounds relatively easy to do. However, like any new skill, mindfulness takes time and practice to hone, particularly when our minds feel busy. For many of those I support, their experiences from the past, and anxieties about the future, mean that they aren't present in the moment. By learning to stay consciously aware of what is happening, being mindful allows them to observe and accept their body, mind, and environmental experiences in the present. This, in turn, provides opportunities to slow down their busy minds, allow more considered decisions, and choose how to respond to what is happening.

Moments of calm can be found in a technique called 7–11 breathing. It does wonders for calming our autonomic nervous system. When we breathe in, we get a burst of adrenaline, and when we breathe out, we relax. Breathing out for longer than the in-breath sends signals automatically to the brain that we are starting to calm. When we begin to relax, the rational thinking part of our brain comes back online.

Unlocking the power of the vagus nerve

Everyone responds differently to stress; what might feel stressful or overwhelming for one person might feel less threatening for another. Although what triggers this response is individual, what happens in everyone's body when they become stressed is the same, thanks to the fantastic role of the vagus nerve.

This nerve is incredibly powerful. It originates in the brain stem and travels throughout our bodies to most of our vital organs. It can process data swiftly, sending impulses

7–11 breathing

To incorporate this into your daily routine, I suggest tagging it on to an existing habit. So, perhaps try it each time you go to make a hot drink, walk down the corridor, before going to see the next woman, or when you sit down to write notes.

- Breathe in, counting to 7, and breath out with a long, slow out-breath, counting to 11.
- Repeat this as often as you like.
- Say something affirming inwardly, or quietly on the out-breath: 'I am calm', 'I am safe', or 'this feeling will pass' – whatever works best to soothe you.

from the body straight to the brain almost instantaneously, without having to travel through the spine, enabling the body to respond rapidly. It has many different roles, regulating the autonomic nervous system, breathing, digestion, inflammation, and mood. It is a wonder nerve!

Toning the vagus nerve, a bit like toning muscles, is one way to ensure it functions optimally. Therefore, it needs to be used daily to enhance its efficiency, and if used less often, its potency will dwindle. When the vagus nerve is toned, the ability to manage difficult emotions is strengthened, enabling individuals to respond differently when faced with an emotionally provocative situation and return to a state of relaxation more quickly afterwards.

Mindfulness is one way to activate the vagus nerve, and below are some other suggestions to stimulate it:

- *Smiling:* The vagus nerve is directly involved in those

parts of the brain and body involved in socialisation. Therefore, smiling can trigger the nerve to activate.

- *Humming/singing:* The vagus nerve passes throughout the vocal chords, through the neck, and into the body. Humming or singing vibrates the vocal chords, activating the nerve, which can feel soothing for some.
- *Laughing:* Everyone knows how to laugh. You can watch something funny, recall a particularly comical memory, anything that makes you laugh.
- *Yoga:* This is a great technique to innervate the vagus nerve as it allows the body to stretch and relax, and involves mindfulness. One or two gentle relaxation poses are suitable for beginners and take a few minutes. You could start with Child's Pose.
- *Cold shower:* The diving reflex functions to shift how the body operates when submerged in water, particularly cold water. It changes the breathing, and the heart rate begins to slow down, in an attempt to restrict blood flow away from the limbs to the essential organs and the brain, because of the vagus nerve. So, triggering the diving reflex can activate the nerve, enabling your body to slow down. At the end of a shower, rinsing with cold water will stimulate this response, or you can splash cold water over your whole face, remembering also to hold your breath. Alternatively, covering your face, especially the forehead and the area around the nose, with a cold, wet towel, will also activate the diving reflex.

Kindness

Kindness is shown in the smallest of acts. For me, it starts with the individual learning how to be kind to themselves. In my experience many people find this challenging to do, as it is usually something they don't typically think about. I love

Beginning to be kind to yourself

I invite you to:

- Think of 2–3 actions that reflect kindness to yourself, such as going to the toilet when you need to, having a drink of water, or having a snack.
- When your mind is loud and being unkind, try to generate self-compassion.

this quote by Maya Angelou: *'If I'm not good to myself, how can I expect anyone else to be good to me?'* to remind us of the need to look after ourselves.

Most people can recall an act of kindness shown to them. Take a moment now to pause, and remember this experience. What immediately comes to my mind was when I gave birth to my first child. Days of labour rendered me utterly exhausted. The night I birthed, a midwife took our baby for a couple of hours while my partner and I got some sleep. I remember awakening in a panic, wondering where my baby was. As I walked down the corridor in the dead of night, I could hear a soft, gentle voice singing, which I followed. As I walked into the room where the singing was coming from, I saw that my baby was tucked into the midwife's scrubs; she was singing to her while writing her notes. That vision of her sitting there with our baby is still so vivid, and her kindness and warmth were a comfort blanket around us all that night.

Acts of kindness don't need to be as grand as that. When I speak with staff about being kind to themselves and others at work, the most common response I hear about why they struggle to show it is, 'we don't have time'.

Kindness is an action. It is a habit we can begin to practise, and it can take as little as a few seconds. For example, some simple yet powerful acts of kindness are:

- The tone of voice when speaking
- Making eye contact with colleagues
- A genuine warm smile
- Saying please and thank you
- Acknowledging the effort colleagues have made on their shift

These all take seconds, but they do require an intention: to *be* kind.

We all can break the cycle of unhelpful patterns we might practise. Kindness is a universal language, which breaks down barriers in our relationships with others. Acts of kindness are contagious, and I have witnessed the domino effect in teams when a couple of people actively choose to be kind. This starts with having the mind-set of wanting to '*be the change we want to see.*' (Gandhi).

Anchor in safety

How do you manage having argued with your partner as you leave for work, the grief of losing a loved one, or having battled to get the kids out of the house, which has now left you running late? Can you turn up to work and 'leave it at the door'? This is incredibly difficult for most of us, and we are rarely taught *how* to do this, even if it is suggested. We bring our whole selves to work.

Anchoring is one way to protect maternity staff when they are feeling heightened levels of stress. The idea of anchoring is a tool used to support clients, particularly in trauma therapy. The technique involves accessing sensory memories that are associated with safety and support. It is effective in shielding from the effects of vicarious trauma, and outlined

Finding your anchor

- Choose a memory, preferably of a place or person. One that makes you feel safe, happy, and calm. Avoid memories associated with tragedy.
- As you connect with the memory, awaken the sensory parts (visual, smells, tastes, tactile, auditory). What do you see? Do you remember any smells or tastes? What can you hear?
- As you recall this memory, what is happening to your body sensations right now? If you notice tension, irritation, or anxiety, perhaps choose a different memory.
- Test it out by remembering a mildly uncomfortable situation from work, and then switch to the calming image of your anchor as soon as you begin to feel uncomfortable.
- Practising switching between difficult memories and your sensory anchors will enable you to access this technique more easily to mediate stress.

here is a way to help find your anchor.[16]

By distilling and refining, a sensory anchor can be used in moments when work begins to feel overwhelming or to help access a calmer state if there is a situation that feels anxiety-provoking.

Seeking support

It is great to see the plethora of campaigns and advertisements now trying to promote the available services to help those requiring emotional and mental support. I hear those I support compare themselves to colleagues who appear unaffected, and the message they've received is that they are struggling because they were not resilient enough, tough enough, thick-skinned enough. It is not because they are not *enough*. It is because human suffering affects everyone at some point in their lives; that is a fact. How we deal with that is individual.

If you would like support, please speak to your GP or another healthcare professional to find out what is available in your area. Many governing bodies that maternity staff are registered with have resources offering support for mental wellbeing.

If you feel you are in crisis because of your current feelings, please seek an urgent appointment with your GP or visit A & E.

Key messages

Changing systems

- Psychologically equip maternity students to work in an emotionally challenging environment.
- Invest in staff wellbeing: financial, resources, and infrastructure.
- Create open and honest cultures.

Promoting wellbeing in teams

- Normalise that difficult emotions are expected working in maternity care.
- Host regular team reflective practice sessions and individual supervision.
- Provide a range of support staff can access when care doesn't go as expected.

Individual wellbeing

Below are some suggestions to help maternity staff maintain mental wellbeing. These are by no means an exhaustive list and are meant to inspire you to create your own.

In 30–90 seconds:
- Smile (to yourself or a colleague)
- 7–11 breathing (see page 99)
- Mindfully, feel your feet on the floor, or your bum in the seat
- Hum/sing to yourself

In five minutes:
- Finding your anchor (see page 103)
- Make a colleague a drink
- Open the window and get some fresh air
- Have a glass of water or a snack

In 30 minutes:
- Have a 15–20-minute nap
- Listen to some music or read
- Watch something funny
- Meditate

6

EMBRACING DIFFERENCE

'There is always light if only we're brave enough to see it. If only we're brave enough to be it.'

Amanda Gorman

In 2020, the world began to wake and question, listen, and take action around diversity, equity, and inclusion, particularly racism, more than ever before. To say this was long overdue is an understatement. Like many of you, I continue to tend to my own personal work with this. I have learned that it requires an open heart, a commitment not to harm others, and fundamentally a willingness to lean into pain and discomfort. This chapter is by no means a blueprint on *how* to do that work, for that is your journey. Instead, it explores what might help or get in the way of turning towards our discomfort and creating a culture of inclusivity within maternity.

Power

If we feel we have it, we have a choice about how we use it. In the leadership programmes and workshops I run for maternity staff, we always consider power: what it is, how it's used, and how to gain feedback from those you lead. I think many of us have a strange relationship with the word *power*. It conjures up lots of different associations. Some of these are positive: empowering, inspirational – whereas others are less so: controlling, forceful. Most of us have experienced what it feels like to be powerless, and it can be an overwhelming and lonely place to be.

Over the years, I have heard countless stories from maternity staff about feeling powerless because of systemic or organisational factors, or because of the behaviours of their colleagues or senior staff. Feeling powerlessness is threatening, and we will have a strong urge to behave in ways that stop us from feeling that way and allow us to regain a sense of control. However, if control isn't restored, this can harm our mental and physical wellbeing. Evidence suggests that those who feel they have little power in their lives have a greater risk of illnesses and death, even when factors like socioeconomic status are controlled for.[1] Power in itself is not an issue; it's how we use it that makes it dangerous to ourselves and others.

Fear is often the driver behind exerting power over people. As previously discussed in Chapter 2, many of you experience fear in your role. That is not to say that all maternity workers turn up to work feeling fearful. Rather, it might be something that is inherently part of your psyche because you have learned that the world does not accept you as equal in some way.

Below are some questions to prompt you to think about your power, how you might use it and what happens when you experience feeling powerless.

Power exercise

- What words come to mind when you think of the word power?
- How might you know you're using your power over others?
- What do you put in place to actively ensure power with another is balanced, even when you are in a more senior position to them?
- What factors impact on you to feel powerless?
- What can you do to feel safe and connected to people who value you at these times?

Language matters

At Make Birth Better, we launched a campaign called #everywordcounts. This campaign acknowledges the power that language and words have in maternity services. Words matter, because they hold power and have the ability to create, or overcome, barriers to connecting with others. The impact of this can be subtle or more obvious.

Over the years, when I've asked staff I'm supporting or training *'What is your name?'*, many have shared their name and then followed this with a shortened or anglicised version, or what their colleagues call them, *'because no one knows how to pronounce my real name'*. I've had the opportunity to explore with many of these people the impact of not being called by their 'real name'. Many have been accepting of it, but others less so, understandably. However, we should recognise that this is a problem: many staff are working in healthcare who accept that they will have to change parts of who they are to make things easier for others.

We can all take time to get to know the name our colleagues prefer to be called by. Also, if you have a name that people initially find difficult to pronounce, rather than default to shortening it to make it easier for them, if you feel able to, you can support them to learn how to say it. It matters that people know the name you want to be called by.

Although there might not be any malice intended, assumptions can wound others, from names and pronouns, to how we learn. Most people are not offended when they can see others making an effort to understand who they are, and how they like to be referred to, so don't feel afraid to ask. We all learn differently and have our own learning style, so when information is explained in a way we can't quite grasp, it isn't exclusively down to the learner to muddle their way through and make sense of the material. It is also the responsibility of the educator to ensure that what is said is received in the way it was intended and the other person has understood because it is a two-way relationship.

When we have learned to change who we are to make it easier for others to accept, this can be deeply wounding. Learning the language of others is not disrespectful: it's the complete opposite. Within teams there will be a diverse range of different histories, experiences, abilities and cultures. We all can create multiple opportunities to understand and learn about one another, with openness and empathy. This fosters connections that are enriching and respectful.

Seeing the person

The latest MBRRACE report[2] stated that in the UK, black women are still four times more likely to die in pregnancy or childbirth, and women from Asian ethnic backgrounds face twice the risk compared to white women. Quite rightly, there are now more focused efforts and investment to address the system biases impacting the care of women from diverse ethnic communities. Of the NHS staff known to have died due to Covid-19, most were black, Asian or from other diverse communities.[3] In response to the disproportionate number ethnic minority people impacted by Covid-19 a review was conducted into the causes of disparities in four areas: health provision, employment, education and criminal justice. These results were published and spoken about in the House of Commons, minimising the impact of institutional and societal racism across Britain, and it was claimed that saying that 'the system is deliberately rigged against ethnic minorities' is no longer the case. However, staff from ethnic minority backgrounds working in the NHS are less likely to be promoted into senior positions, face greater barriers to career progression, are more likely to enter formal disciplinary processes, and experience more harassment, bullying and abuse from colleagues, patients and their relatives than their white colleagues.[4,5] The tragedy is that many of these differences and gaps are getting worse, not better.[5,6] The recent publication of the NHS People Plan acknowledges shortcomings in inclusion and diversity in the NHS, and sets out ways to address this. While this is a welcome step, the attitudes, beliefs and behaviours that result in many NHS staff experiencing discrimination, racism, marginalisation and abuse urgently needs addressing.

Statistics help to gain an understanding on the gravity of the situation, but nonetheless they fall short in giving us a full picture. As harrowing as the figures are, there's a danger that we lose sight of the people behind the statistics: their stories, their experiences.

A thread that runs throughout this book is the importance of relationships; with ourselves, our colleagues, and the women, birthing people and families we support. Developing and maintaining these relationships doesn't always happen, and this has far-reaching negative consequences. Empathy is the glue to enable connections with others. When we lose our empathy, not only does this hurt those we are trying to support in our roles, but we hurt ourselves too. A loss of empathy for others can often be symptomatic of high levels of compassion fatigue. Additionally, we all have internal attitudes and stereotypes that affect our actions, understanding, and decisions, and we're not usually even aware of them (this is known as implicit or unconscious bias).

At the centre of relational interactions is empathy, making it possible for staff to be valued, listened to, and accepted. Creating empathy and trust is essential for people to feel safe. This can happen when we are aware of our biases, work to change them, and look for opportunities to be curious and empathic with colleagues. I previously discussed the importance of psychological safety within teams. While this is crucial for *everyone* to feel heard, respected, and valued, we all have a responsibility to ensure that interactions we have with our colleagues are safe too.

Many things might interfere with empathising with another and 'seeing' the person who stands before you, not for what they represent, but for the human being they are. For example, empathising with someone else requires us to connect with a part of ourselves that is vulnerable and can relate to that person's experience. It sounds simple to do, doesn't it? But if, for whatever reason, you are unable to connect with yourself, either because it's too painful, threatening, or unsafe, it might make it more difficult for you to empathise with another. Additionally, empathising with others means we need to create a space in our heads and hearts where we can 'hold' their experience. If you're burnt out, feeling high levels of compassion fatigue or experiencing trauma-related symptoms, this will compromise your ability to empathise with others. I want to be clear; I am not making excuses for unacceptable behaviours. Instead, we need to understanding the context in which unkind, toxic, and intimidating behaviours exist.

Our prejudices, judgements, stigmas, and stereotypes can not only cloud how we see others we perceive as being different from ourselves, but they can also sever our connections and magnify divisions within organisations. It is not for me to dictate to others the self-development work they should do: that is a personal choice. Over my time working alongside maternity staff, I've learned a fundamental lesson. For maternity services to be safe for staff, women, and families, it takes an effort from everyone: chief executives, senior leaders, managers, clinical and non-clinical staff. There needs to be a shared vision on what the maternity service should be and the values that underpin it. It needs to be explicitly made clear what the behaviours are that demonstrate these commitments, and all staff, at every level, are accountable when it comes to upholding them.

Accountability isn't, nor should it be, threatening or confrontational. It is a safety net to hold everyone engaged in a shared vision and goal – ensuring that staff and users of maternity services feel emotionally, psychologically, and physically safe. Making changes in our beliefs, attitudes, values, and behaviours is complex and can undoubtedly be painful. For organisations it can be challenging to know where to start. It can begin with providing the space to listen to what staff need in a way that breaks down their armour. This can and has been achieved by organisations that have successfully created this by fostering compassion, kindness, and respect.

Slowing the pace

Rarely is self-development work something that can be completed quickly and ticked off the list as a 'job done'. That's a bit like saying that when you meet someone new for the first time, and have a few more interactions with them, then a week later you know them in a deep and meaningful way. The relationship we have with ourselves is one in which we learn, reflect, and evolve. This won't always feel like we're moving forward; rarely are relationships a smooth ride, and the relationship with ourselves is no different.

However, when we are moved to action, as many of us have been, particularly around racism, there might be an urgency to act. While the motivation behind this is more than likely well-intended, it also highlights the disparity, because it has required action long ago. Action bias describes our desire to lean towards action over inaction, which often benefits us in some way. Being able to slow down, be present and listen to those we wish to support is a privileged position many of us hold. We can use this positively and productively to work collaboratively and make long-lasting changes.

When we're on a train journey, it's not often we see the detail of the landscape because the train is travelling so fast. When we rush to act, for example, because of our own discomfort, or we need to 'be seen' to be doing something, we won't capture the experiences of those we need to work with and for. Maternity services are fast-paced: things happen quickly, and so many staff are primed to act when they are alerted. Overriding the desire to fix, slow down, see the person, and create the space for change to happen is something many have to learn how to do.

This requires us to actively look out for opportunities to slow the pace and create space for change. It could be in the interactions with those we perceive as different in some way to ourselves and the moments between those interactions. Sonya Renée Taylor is an inspiring transformational leader, and author of *The Body is Not an Apology: The Power of Radical Self-Love*. She shares three key pieces of learning for us all: making peace with not understanding, making peace with difference, and making peace with your body. This isn't possible to do when we pursue a 'quick fix' solution. Rather it's noticing the feelings that arise in us and any judgements, criticisms, words our minds are saying. Not just for the select few, but for us all, we're all in it.

Below is a fictitious scenario between June and Beth. There are two different responses from June. In one, she actively looks for opportunities to connect, learn about, and value Beth, and in the other, she doesn't.

Beth is a third-year student midwife who is black. She has arranged to meet with her mentor June, a white midwife, to discuss some feedback she received about a birth she assisted with. Beth shared that the colleague she assisted, Rachel, had spoken harshly to her in front of their other colleagues, and she didn't really understand what she had done wrong.

Response 1
June could see that Beth was upset by what had happened. June responded, 'I'm sorry you're upset, it's a steep learning curve, and it's probably better that you got that feedback now before you qualified. This is part of your learning, and it will help to build up your resilience. She probably didn't mean anything by it. You

know what Rachel's like.'

Beth left June's office feeling worse than she did before she went in.

Response 2
June could see that Beth was upset by what had happened.

June: [Opportunity to understand Beth's experience].
    'Tell me a little more about what happened?'

Beth: *'I'm not quite sure – the delivery seemed to have gone fine. I did everything I was asked to. We got back to the office, and I shared with the others how well the birth had gone. I felt pleased with it all. Rachel tutted when I said this and said to our colleagues about how slowly I had been doing everything and that if I was going to make it as a midwife, I needed to be much faster. She then said people like me were always slower, and when I qualified, I wouldn't have the luxury of time. She didn't even look at me.'*

June: [Opportunity to connect with Beth, her experience, understand more, and empathise].
    'That sounds like a really difficult experience, standing there in front of all your colleagues and Rachel speaking about you in that way. How was that for you?'

Beth: *'I was confused and still am about what I did. I felt humiliated and embarrassed. I didn't know what to say, and no one else said anything. They just went back to their work, and I was left standing there in the middle of the office, not really knowing what to do.'*

June: [Opportunity to empathise with Beth, ensure she feels believed and valued, and that she is supported]. *'That sounds like such a painful experience for you, Beth. I'm sorry you had to go through that, and it shouldn't have happened. It might not be the time to do this now, but I wonder how it might be for you to think about ways to address this and what you might need from me. We can do this together, or I can support you to do this, whatever you think will be most helpful to you.'*

In the first response, June has missed the multiple opportunities to connect with Beth, demonstrate empathy and create a space where she feels believed and heard. In the second response, which requires time, June can connect with something in herself to be able to empathise with Beth. She doesn't assume that Rachel's behaviour was acceptable, she believes Beth's experience and she doesn't rush her to create a solution to how June might best support her.

Creating nurturing cultures

Generally, the culture within healthcare is perceived as the softer and less tangible aspect of services. Yet culture has been cited as contributing to many historic failings in healthcare.[4] There are many parts of maternity services that are great and work well. So, when changing a culture, it isn't necessarily radically overhauling all of it, but identifying the parts that aren't working well and actively changing or erasing them.

Although creating a positive working culture starts with leaders, you don't need to be in a leadership position to contribute. This can be done in the hundreds of daily interactions you have with colleagues. Most organisations have several subcultures, and the power of these can force positive changes, or conversely, sabotage quality improvements, which makes changing a culture potentially complex. As I've mentioned before, we bring our whole selves to work, our histories and experiences are interwoven into the fabric of our being. Because of this, the culture in which we work can then act to nurture or wound us. Let me explain a little more.

As humans, we have a stress response, which I wrote about in Chapter 1. It's essential to keep us safe, and most of the time it does a great job of this. However, if growing up you were perceived and treated by others in a way which activated your stress response, then you might have learned that the world was unsafe and you then behaved in ways that helped you feel safer. This might have continued into adulthood. Therefore, in daily interactions with others and environments you navigate, if you experience a behaviour, a look, a gesture, a comment that tells you that you're different in some way, this will activate your stress response. Over time, if this prolonged, it can lead to changes in the brain that are the same as if you had experienced a significant traumatic event, like a car accident or serious assault.

These past and present experiences will result in a heightened stress response and you might learn that keeping your 'armour' on is not a choice, but a necessity to survive. Therefore, you might engage in behaviours that keep you guarded and protected, but that don't necessarily serve you to be the person that you truly want to be. If this is the case for you, it can be helpful to talk it through with someone you trust, in order to:

- Understand why these behaviours exist
- Identify what no longer serves you well
- Let these behaviours go in a way that feels safe for you

The brain is one of the most incredible and fascinating organs. Working in neuropsychology for many years, I witnessed the amazing ability our brains have to repair and build new pathways. As humans, we are built to socialise and connect with other people. The field of trauma research has demonstrated that when we are in the presence of others who make us feel safe, that we belong, and that we are valued, this can have a profound effect on healing and recovery from trauma. Our stress response systems become more regulated and the reward systems in our brain are stimulated. This reduces the need to engage in less helpful adaptive behaviours, like alcohol and drug use, to get those rewards. Imagine the potential power of our daily interactions, in which we all have the ability to help those we work with and support feel seen and included. Maternity services could be a place of nurture and healing not only for the staff working in them, but for those who use these services too.

Given that unpredictability and feeling like we have a lack of control can activate our stress responses, maternity services can potentially buffer the impact of this on staff by being 'trauma informed'. There isn't a checklist of what to do to create a trauma informed service, rather it requires sensitivity, constant attention, and awareness to create a place where *everyone* feels safe and can trust those around them. Undoubtedly this will require a culture shift by leaders who are compassionate, transparent and are able to empower those they lead.

If you are working in maternity and experience yourself as being in the 'out group' within an 'in culture', think about ways that support you to feel safe in your interactions with others. Also, in Chapter 5 there are suggestions about ways to respond when faced with stressors that allow your stress response to return to a state of relaxation much more quickly. Having boundaries, for example areas of your life that you won't discuss at work, and feeling comfortable exercising these boundaries, will serve to emotionally protect you.

As an individual, a team, or an organisation, it might be that creating a safe, diverse and inclusive culture is being considered, has already started, or is well underway. It will never be complete because it is always an ongoing process. The example below is from someone who shared their experience.

'I had prepared myself to go to work and get some questions because the programme about transgender people had been aired the night before. I started my shift, and within the first half an hour, three of my colleagues had asked me which pronoun I would prefer to be called by. While I appreciated their sentiment, it felt very uncomfortable. Another person asked me directly "which bits of my body did I still have left". I went into work as a midwife, not as an educator on transgender people, language to use, or the process involved. It's not that I was offended necessarily. I know what it's like to deal with being different. It's more that it wasn't safe for me to get into those conversations at my workplace. No one ever asked me any of these questions before the programme. If they did, I might have been more inclined to have the conversation. It felt more like they'd watched a programme and thought, "we've got one of those [transgender people] in our team, I must do something". I felt pretty violated actually, like my boundaries were being trampled all over.'

Anonymous

As the person in this example demonstrated, we can work in places with a diverse range of people, but if they don't feel safe and included, diversity becomes a tick-box exercise. If you are an individual who feels different in some way, it is not down to you to educate colleagues. If this is something that you want to do, it should be done in a way that you feel comfortable with, and with boundaries in place to safeguard you. Also you should be remunerated in some way for the knowledge, experience and expertise you have in teaching others.

Therefore, it is not enough to just create environments where everyone can express how they feel and share ideas. It is imperative that when people do this, they feel respected, valued and that their experience matters. NHS Trusts all tend to have a Diversity, Equity, and Inclusion policy nowadays. Each time we don't define the meaning of these to staff, and the behaviours expected to reflect them, staff from diverse backgrounds continue to be at risk of being emotionally and psychologically wounded in the workplace.

We all have the power not to harm those we work with. This will always be an ongoing process for individuals and at an organisational level. For any change to occur, this has to be relational, where we connect with others, their experiences, and the person they are. At the heart of this is a psychologically safe culture, in which staff are valued, respected, and celebrated for who they are. This involves self-development work individually but also collectively, leaning in to the inevitable discomfort in the service of making maternity services nurturing places for all.

7

DARE TO DREAM

'It is never too late to be what you might have been.'
George Eliot

Hope. By its very definition, it is future-orientated. Situations staff find themselves in can feel hopeless, and this might feel all-consuming at times. Yet, when aspects of our lives feel dark, and when tomorrow looks grim, the embers of hope are what need stoking so we can find faith that the situation will change.

Much of my work is supporting those who are psychologically wounded and their spirit broken. Creating meaning in their present and hope for their future is an integral part of my role. Whether or not a system thrives is not down to the building or the equipment it houses. It's down to the people within it. Therefore, consciously creating spaces where all staff can be human is essential if they are to feel valued and perform the job they are trained to do. There are some excellent maternity services across the UK, where staff are valued and supported, which ultimately helps them care compassionately. A consensus among women and staff is that maternity services have to change for the better. This chapter sets out a vision for how maternity services could be. Each person who has contributed their wisdom and experiences in this chapter is a purveyor of hope: that maternity can be a better experience for everyone.

Sufficient resources

Each year the NHS Staff Survey collates responses to questions about levels of staff satisfaction with workplace conditions. In 2019 less than one-third of staff across all NHS sectors reported positive action on health and wellbeing in their organisation, adequate staffing to enable them to do their jobs properly, and senior staff who act on their feedback. In the past year, up to 45% felt unwell due to work-related stress, and 25% of respondents were making plans to leave the organisation within 12 months.[1] This was before the Covid-19 pandemic hit.

Having sufficient staffing levels is vital to ensure that women receive quality care. Given the levels of mental health difficulties in staff, psychological injuries inflicted on women, and soaring litigation costs, ensuring there are enough staff, and that they are fairly paid, needs addressing as a matter of urgency. Staff also need adequate equipment to carry out their jobs as safely as possible.

Chapter 4 discussed the Camden Coalition of Healthcare Providers in New Jersey, which invested in staff wellbeing, encouraging self-care practices and accessing mental health support services. Staff have repeatedly shared with me that although they appreciate the sentiment, receiving an email reminder to drink more water or attend a yoga class doesn't constitute a genuine investment in their wellbeing. Looking after oneself, first and foremost, should be valued and modelled by the organisation's leaders to facilitate a culture change. Investment in adequate staffing levels is also an investment in staff wellbeing. Time is precious for staff in the NHS because they want more of it but can't get it. So, when anything threatens an already time-poor organisation, staff will understandably fight to cling to whatever time they have. Having sufficient staff and resources distributes the workload more equally, which contributes to staff feeling less overworked. Feeling valued in work is a foreign experience for many or a distant memory. Staff are taught as students to provide compassionate maternity care, but they rarely are taught *how* to thrive at work in the NHS. If leaders, senior maternity officials, and government ministers all worked collaboratively to foster maternity services that were safe, caring, nurturing, and kind places to provide *and* receive care, the positive effect could be immense.

Maternity environments are psychologically safe

The importance of creating psychologically safe working environments for staff was discussed in Chapter 2. This ensures they feel able to speak out about whatever they think is important and that in doing so, they are met with openness, affirmation, and curiosity from their colleagues. Professor Rebecca Lawton, the Director of NIHRR Yorkshire and Humber Patient Safety Translational Research Centre, and Dr Tomasina Stacey, Associate Professor of Midwifery Practice, share their vision of what psychological safety could be in maternity services.

> *'Imagine that you arrive on shift, and you are feeling a bit unsure of yourself after a difficult shift the week before when one of the women you supported sustained a third-degree tear. Today you know you will be working with a new team leader (coordinator) who you have never met before. Before the shift starts, the team "huddles", and the new coordinator introduces herself and says*

that her main goal is to make sure everyone on her shift feels psychologically safe. At the end of the shift, you feel lighter and that you have been able to be yourself a bit more. The shift has been busy and challenging, but you felt able to be honest when you were unsure about how to interpret certain clinical findings, you felt supported to ask questions when you worried about the decision of a senior doctor, and you were encouraged to speak up and offer a solution when there was a problem with equipment availability. This is what psychological safety feels like.

So, what exactly is psychological safety, and why is it so important? First described by Kahn in 1990 and then further refined by Amy Edmondson,[2] psychological safety is best defined as "a shared belief that the team is safe for interpersonal risk taking".

To better understand what a psychologically safe culture would look like, it is helpful to consider some of the questionnaire items used to measure the extent to which it exists in teams. There are many measures of psychological safety, but they consistently include items such as the following from Edmondson:[3]

- *If you make a mistake on this team, it is often held against you –*
- *Members of this team are able to bring up problems and tough issues +*
- *People on this team sometimes reject others for being different –*
- *It is safe to take a risk on this team +*
- *It is difficult to ask other members of this team for help –*
- *No one on this team would deliberately act in a way*

that undermines my efforts +
- *Working with members of this team, my unique skills and talents are valued and utilized +*

If you answer yes to all the questions marked by a +sign and no to those marked with a -sign, you probably work in a team with high levels of psychological safety. This is important because recent research findings and other evidence have found that psychological safety in teams is related to work satisfaction, patient safety, productivity, and a whole range of different positive outcomes.

A large study of team performance by Google[4] involving interviews with more than 200 staff and assessment of 180 teams found that the strongest factor that underpinned team success was psychological safety. Within Google, this might mean having a crazy idea and feeling able to talk about it or asking for clarification of the goal of a task without being made to feel stupid. While the context of maternity is different, some things are the same. We are human, so we want to be liked, perceived as competent, and not a trouble causer. As Riskin[5] and others have shown in healthcare settings, the way we speak to each other can affect teamwork: lack of civility impacts psychological safety. These basic human needs can, in a psychologically unsafe team, lead to ineffective teamwork.

For example, the recent Each Baby Counts[6] report highlights issues with escalation and handover as critically important and identifies psychological safety as paramount in ensuring patient safety. The report discusses the advantages of flattened hierarchies:

"It removes the assumption that the decision of the

most senior doctor or midwife is final and promotes an environment of psychological safety for staff to speak up, challenge seniors when needed, and request a second opinion without repercussions."

Supporting and caring for women through pregnancy and birth involves emotional work and clinical work.[7] Psychological safety within this context is therefore of particular relevance. A psychologically safe culture is where all team members feel supported rather than scrutinised, where they feel seen and heard, and where attention is paid to what is communicated and how it is communicated.'

Healing when care doesn't go as expected

In healthcare, mistakes are sometimes made. This is a sad fact for both the patient and staff involved. The ripple effect when care doesn't go as expected can be life-changing. As well as providing therapy, I carry out psychological assessments as an expert witness for families who have been involved in maternity incidents where care did not go as expected. In understanding countless families' experiences over the years, it is clear that their need to pursue litigation action is often motivated by not wanting another family to go through what happened to them, and a desire for an apology or recognition of what has happened. It would seem that the 'duty of candour' would cover this: staff have a legal duty to be open and honest with patients/families when potential or significant harm has been caused. However, this is often not the case.

Imagine how different things would be in cases of potential or actual harm if families and the staff involved were offered psychological support for as long as they needed it. This would also help facilitate a meeting between the staff involved and the family, and the events that led to the care not going as planned could be discussed openly and honestly. Changes to help prevent the same incident occurring in the future could then be implemented (and reviewed). Finally, a heartfelt and sincere apology could be made. This won't change what has happened and remove the emotional pain felt, but I have witnessed the power this process can have for healing those wounded. Michelle Hemmington, from the Campaign for Safer Births, shares her experience:

'When our son died unexpectedly due to failings in care throughout my labour and his birth, we were submerged into a world we never knew existed. I think I was so shrouded in shock and disbelief that I couldn't process what had happened at first. The grief was one I had never experienced before, and everything felt alien and unreal. Throughout the hospital investigation and subsequent legal process, it felt very much like "us and them". We had gone from trusting the staff that were supposed to have been looking after us to not seeing or hearing from them again. This in itself was very difficult as we never knew if they were sorry for what had happened or had learned from his death or not. I just wanted to know they were sorry. I think this would have made a difference to the grieving process and the anger we felt.'

For Michelle and many others in her situation, having the opportunity to meet with those involved would undoubtedly have helped in her grief. In the absence of families and staff being given a chance to share, understand, and learn, toxic emotions can manifest. This can prolong or sabotage the healing process.

Leila Benyounes, a specialist clinical negligence barrister, has this to say about representing families and staff where care has not gone as expected:

'*Many women have a different birth experience from what they expected, and sadly cases of birth trauma have apparent similarities. In cases I have been involved in, repeated themes are feelings of a loss of control and mothers stating that they did not feel that they were being listened to. In many cases, key information was only provided after the event following internal investigations, as part of the inquest process, or as part of a clinical negligence claim.*

It should not be forgotten that genuine efforts have already been made to improve maternity services. Communication goes a long way to improving a birth experience, like compassion, kindness, recognition of mistakes, and acceptance of errors without fear of repercussion. It is a long journey.'

Diversity, inclusion, and equality in maternity care

We have an opportunity in the UK to make genuine changes to ensure that staff in maternity services are not just diverse, but also that the workspaces they occupy are inclusive. This means that it is psychologically and physically safe for *all* staff, irrespective of their race, gender, sexual or religious orientation, culture, disabilities, learning abilities, neurodiversity and mental and physical challenges, to be the person they are and valued. To create this in the workplace is a huge task, and I don't have the answers to this. However, I know it requires us to listen with an open heart, an open mind, and a willingness to connect with discomfort in ourselves and those around us. Leaders have a crucial role in paving the way for what it means to have true diversity, inclusion, and equality in maternity.

Benash Nazmeen, specialist cultural liaison midwife, shared her vision of cultural diversity and equality within maternity services. She dared to dream.

'Race can be defined as each of the significant groupings into which humankind is considered (in various theories or contexts) to be divided on the basis of physical characteristics or shared ancestry.

Another definition for race is a competition between runners, horses, vehicles, etc., to see which is the fastest in covering a set course.

In reality, a fair, competitive race considers the starting line and often has a strict just criterion for eligibility. This is what one expects; however, the reality is in the race for life in the UK, there is a disparity between ethnicities.[8,9,10]

This racial injustice within maternity services hasn't been addressed as all the reports and research avoid using one term that is part of the multifactorial issues that lead to this disparity.

Racism has been termed bias; unconscious bias, implicit bias to be more palatable. The systemic issues have descended from historical racism, and to address an issue we have to accept and name it first.

I dream of a day when healthcare professionals can openly discuss this issue, name it and work towards addressing it, individually, together, and systemically. I dream of a day when ethnically diverse communities are believed when they raise these issues, rather than being asked to prove or example it. The trauma this triggers *and the distrust it builds just adds to the barriers faced by these communities, and this is causing harm.*

I dream of a day when representation of diversity is across the board, without tokenism, with a focus on equity. As those with lived experience who have overcome their internalised racism can identify and highlight needs of the communities, so we do not fail them again.

I dream of the day when we treat people as individuals, not a label or an acronym, to make our lives easier. When staff respect individuals enough to learn how to pronounce their names without anglicising or shortening.

I dream of a day when the interview and application processes for university and work are fair and unbiased. Where we can have increased representation within the workforce of the communities we care for.

I dream of a day when the educational gap in learning is addressed when we remove the Eurocentric lens from our teaching and apply context of history to the discoveries. When the materials we read have representative images, authors and cover the needs of diverse communities. Where the academic staff reflect that representation.

I dream that, like feminism, we can accept racism is a problem without being defensive or uncomfortable to discuss it. Just because you have the privilege of ignorance doesn't mean that you invalidate the experience of another. If you can accept you have picked up unconscious and implicit bias, you should reflect on its historical racist origins.

I dream of a day when we all take the stance of anti-racism because not participating in it is not enough.'

Culture of nurturing for staff

Valuing maternity students

As discussed throughout this book, the impact of burnout, stress and vicarious trauma on student maternity staff is overwhelming, with many leaving their profession shortly after qualifying or changing specialisms. Imagine a maternity system where all students were consistently respected and valued. Apart from the skills and knowledge developed, their passion and curiosity could be embraced and opportunities created, which enabled this to flourish and grow.

Billie Hunter, Professor of Midwifery and director of the WHO Collaborating Centre for Midwifery Development, and Dr Lucie Warren from Cardiff University discuss how to harbour and 'hold' maternity students to ensure they remain in their profession and are psychologically healthy and happy in their work.

'Proactive, compassionate, and sensitive support for midwifery students is essential! It is very difficult to get a place on a UK midwifery education programme, so it's crucial that we offer the best support we can to the students to keep them on the course and make sure they graduate as skilful, thoughtful, and caring midwives. It's important that they appreciate that the course will be a very challenging one, with a demanding academic workload of lectures and assessments alongside clinical learning. When students go into clinical practice, they are exposed to the realities of the work of a midwife from Day One. Ideally, they would have a gentle introduction, but maternity care is unpredictable, and we cannot guarantee that students won't witness a distressing situation. But what we can ensure is that they will receive sensitive and compassionate support, both from the academic teaching team and from their Practice Supervisors and Assessors. And that they feel welcomed into the midwifery 'family', where they'll be surrounded by staff who have passion for their work and a shared vision and voice.

As educators, we need to ensure that students are prepared for the tough realities of working in the NHS. This statement may feel counter-intuitive – surely we want the students to hold on to their ideals? However, we've learned that in order for students to flourish and thrive, they need to be able to anticipate which situations might prove challenging and develop positive coping strategies. Some strategies will be needed at the time of the challenge to help with immediate coping, while others will focus more on coping in the long term.

In order to embed this approach, we have integrated 'resilience' discussions throughout the programme at Cardiff University. These emphasise the importance of developing emotional awareness, both of personal emotions and those of colleagues, to create emotionally safe workspaces. The sessions take the form of workshops which introduce students to theories of psychological wellbeing and the related research, followed by regular small-group tutorials focused on coping in real-life adversity. The emphasis in all these sessions is on building trust and compassion – self-compassion and compassion for others – and mutual respect and kindness. The sessions not only create a safe space where students can share their experiences with peers so that they realise that they are not alone; they also enable students and lecturers to work together to model a supportive and emotionally safe work culture. In all these sessions, we aim to ensure *that students recognise that many adverse situations they encounter will need systemic solutions; it's very important that they don't feel responsible as individuals.*

Our ideas are informed by our study of midwifery resilience.[11] The study recommended that midwifery education should pay attention to "the importance of developing self-awareness and protective self-care, valuing professional identity, and the critical moments in a midwife's career when additional support is needed".[11] We developed a Resilient Repertoire from the study findings,[12] which acts as a prompt for reflection and discussion.

A supportive environment can promote a sense of belonging that encourages empathy and connection with colleagues. We recognised from our research that social support was highly valued when individuals experienced adversity and interestingly that this was equally valued by those giving support as well as those receiving it. In order to promote this peer support within our students, we developed the 'sister scheme'. The sister scheme encourages students to reach out to each other and provide informal support. Similar to the idea of mentoring, this scheme teams up a new first-year student at the start of their studies with a more experienced second-year student. This support continues through the programme so that when students progress to the next academic year, they have support from their 'big sister' as well as providing support to a 'little sister'. Thus ensuring that they are able to both receive and provide support as required. In order to promote autonomy and ownership of the scheme, it is managed by student representatives who pair up the 'sisters'. Students have reported that the sister scheme has assisted those at the start of their training to feel welcomed and part of the midwifery community and facilitated their progression through the programme, building confidence with second-year students eager to take on the role of the supportive 'big sister'.

We recognise that appropriate support of students' progression through the midwifery programme through methods such as the resilience discussions and the sister scheme is of value in fostering a safe and supportive environment, with the aim of increasing wellbeing and lowering attrition of our students. Not only is reducing student attrition important, but increasing retention of newly qualified staff has also been highlighted as a significant area for development.[13] Our research noted that there were key moments in a career when midwives were especially vulnerable to adversity, with recent qualification being identified as one such time. The transition period between being a final year student and taking up employment as a midwife is understood to be especially challenging. In order to tackle this, Approved Education Institutes (AEIs) and Practice Partners across Wales developed the "pre-qualifying placement agreement". The idea behind this is for students to have their final placement within the organisation where they will be employed upon qualification. The purpose of this is threefold: to help their adjustment to the clinical area, enable them to integrate into the midwifery workforce, and assist them in building their confidence while still being supported as a final-year student. We have found that this has enabled a smoother transition to being qualified midwives.

Throughout the programme, we are influenced by the Compassionate Leadership approach developed by

Professor Michael West, which provides such important insights into what is needed to keep NHS staff motivated and engaged.[1] He identifies three core needs which must be attended to if staff are to flourish and thrive:

- *Autonomy – control over work life, and able to behave in a way that is congruent with personal values.*
- *Belonging – feeling connected to colleagues, valued and cared for.*
- *Contribution – feeling effective at work and able to do what matters.[14]*

We aim to keep these core needs central to our thinking as we nurture our students to be the best midwives they can be.'

Compassionate workplaces

Compassion is central to the vast majority of staff working in maternity services. Leaders must lead with compassion to ensure that compassionate cultures are created, not only so that staff provide high-quality, compassionate care, but also so that they show compassion to themselves and their colleagues. By empowering staff at every level to make necessary improvements, leaders should create high levels of trust within the organisation, focusing on minimising hierarchical structures, bureaucracy, and discrimination against minority groups. We don't necessarily need to be in a senior position to be a leader. Everyone can be a leader, championing, advocating, and promoting some part of maternity care. Dr Sally Pezaro, midwifery lecturer and researcher, shares her views on the importance of creating compassionate workplaces in maternity:

'Through all of the research activities I have engaged in, the evidence remains unwavering on the importance of securing psychologically safe professional journeys for maternity staff.[15,16,17] This is particularly important in the pursuit of safer and more effective healthcare services. We know that many midwives still experience work-related psychological distress. Some of this is a result of bullying and trauma. In response, some can display symptomatic behaviours of ill health and/or employ maladaptive coping strategies, neither of which are conducive to safety nor excellence in maternity services.

Doctors have bespoke practitioner health programmes to support them both anonymously and confidentially. Midwives are not afforded the same. On the contrary, our mixed-methods systematic review[18] revealed a lack of evidence-based interventions to support midwives and student midwives in work-related psychological distress. We also know that some midwives presently feel unable to seek support due to the fear, shame, and stigma they may face in response to what some may see as a failure of character. Others are simply leaving the profession altogether. Due to lack of disclosures, we may not even know how deep the rabbit hole may go or how evidence-based bespoke support services may take shape.

One thing we can do to improve the staff experience in maternity services is to demonstrate workplace compassion. This is not rocket science, as our #ShowsWorkplaceCompassion campaign has shown. I have contributed to this book as I felt it would be a safe space to share my own story, insights, and research. I believe we are now at a crucial juncture at which we can either act defensively and be reluctant to address the *issues we face as a profession, or act decisively to unearth and address them wholly, without blame or judgement for what has come before. Despite having come face to face with the internal bullying cultures apparent in the midwifery profession, even while battling my ill health, I now dare to dream again. If we are looking for excellence in maternity services, we must start with the flourishment of midwives. This begins with the start of some uncomfortable conversations and the courage of daring to dream.'*

Trauma-informed services

Adverse Childhood Experiences (ACEs) are potentially traumatic events that occur in childhood and can include violence, abuse, and growing up in a family with mental health or substance misuse problems. Experiencing a higher number of ACEs in childhood can be associated with an increased risk of physical and emotional difficulties across the lifespan.[19] In the UK, one in four people will experience mental illness every year.[20] Given that over one million people work for the NHS, it is likely that many of them will have experienced adverse and potentially traumatising events in their life. Therefore, creating a trauma-informed healthcare system would be advantageous for staff and patients.

Trauma-informed care doesn't mean trauma-specific care, and it doesn't propose to heal or even directly address the trauma. It does involve the whole workforce, from cleaners, receptionists, clinicians and allied professionals being trauma-informed. That means everyone follows four fundamental principles:

1. *Realise* the prevalence of traumatic events and the widespread impact of trauma

2. *Recognise* the signs and symptoms of trauma
3. *Respond* by integrating knowledge about trauma into policies, procedures, and practices, and
4. seek to actively *Resist Re-traumatisation*

The TIC pyramid[21] below can support staff to apply these principles to their organisations.

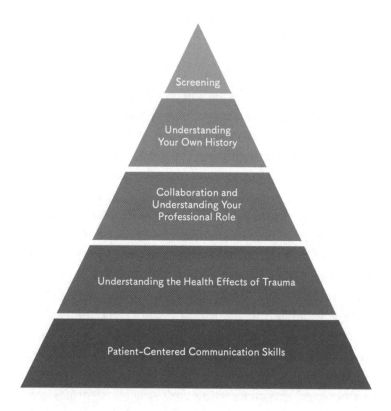

Screening

Understanding Your Own History

Collaboration and Understanding Your Professional Role

Understanding the Health Effects of Trauma

Patient-Centered Communication Skills

Trauma Informed Care Pyramid.

These principles and applications are not exclusively to support the women that staff care for; the trauma-informed environment can also serve to help those who work in it. Dr Jenny Patterson, a midwifery lecturer and researcher from Edinburgh Napier University, discusses how trauma-informed services can impact maternity staff:

'The term *salutogenesis* refers to a scholarly focus on the origins of health, sometimes considered as a focus on the creation of health. In other words, the creation of systems and environments that foster health and enable individuals to thrive and maintain wellbeing. The important and growing focus on trauma-informed care reflects an approach that is about creating wellbeing not by treating issues, but by avoiding creating or exacerbating issues in the first place. In order for midwives and other maternity care providers to truly provide trauma-informed care, they need to be supported in a trauma-informed way and to have their own human needs recognised and met. The statistic of one in four that represents the likelihood of a history of sexual trauma or adverse childhood events[22] applies equally to maternity care providers.

Therefore, if we want to provide compassionate, woman-centred care, we need first to ensure we create compassionate, midwife-centred organisations. Such organisations would ensure that each maternity care provider and manager, at every level, is empowered and supported to thrive. This would include being and feeling welcome within the community of staff; having appropriate rest, hydration, and nutrition; having a safe space to reflect and debrief about experiences; being fully supported in skills and competency development; and zero-tolerance towards undermining and bullying *behaviour.*

Another way to look at this is to explore the ideologies of care known as "Vigil of Care" and "Care as Gift".[23] Vigil of Care can be understood as a top-down management of care provided by the "expert" where risk is monitored and addressed, which often fails to see the personhood of the individual receiving care. In contrast, Care as Gift, while still aiming for safety and reduction of risk, approaches care with generosity, compassion, and even love. Care as Gift is provided within a trustful relationship in which the personhood of the individual is fully acknowledged and respected. Imagine the difference it would make to midwives and all staff in the maternity services if their interactions with one another and those they care for aligned with the ideology of Care as Gift.

Trauma-informed care needs to begin at the very beginning, with each and every staff member in the maternity system. This way, they will be fully enabled to provide the compassionate, skilled, and safe care that they strongly desire to give and thus fulfil the passion and motivation that brought them into this profession in the first place.'

Every day, people who work in maternity services play a vital role in bringing life to the world and giving women and birthing people a sense of security when they might be feeling vulnerable. A sense of life and of being while vulnerable also belongs to each person in the team. The suggestions in this chapter about how maternity services could better care for staff, which in turn would benefit patients, are not borne from naivety or grandiose thinking. Rather, an openness to listen, learn, and the hope that all staff could work in safe, supportive, and nourishing organisations.

Blueprint for maternity services

1. Sufficient resources
2. Psychologically safe culture
3. Healing when care hasn't gone as expected
4. Diversity, Inclusion, and Equality embedded at every level
5. Valuing students
6. Compassionate workplaces
7. Trauma-informed service

CONCLUSION

The year 2020 brought momentous events, which hopefully will positively change those who use and work in maternity services. Some of these events have shone a spotlight on the health inequalities those from Black, Asian and other diverse ethnic communities experience in maternity care, while the global Covid-19 pandemic has highlighted the huge responsibility healthcare staff bear. The Ockenden review focused on safety within maternity services. It was also the global Year of the Nurse and Midwife to celebrate all that our nursing and midwifery colleagues do.

I wholeheartedly believe we can all change. I don't mean that in a soft, fluffy way; in fact, it is the opposite. To change how we behave first requires us to look at ourselves. Not just the parts that are easy to look at, but those parts that are messy, uncontained, and not always comfortable. This is by no means for the faint-hearted: it takes a considerable amount of courage. More than that, it takes a willingness. A willingness to want to be different, to (re)connect with ourselves, others, our passions, our work. Change takes time, and it takes patience. It doesn't have to be completed in one single action; relatively small, considered, and deliberate acts of change can often have the most significant impact.

I hope you have picked up this book because some part of you seeks change in maternity services, and you hope for a different future. You might not even have been aware of it, but reading this book might be the first step in beginning that journey, to be the best version of yourself you can be. I wonder what your next step might be.

CONTRIBUTORS

Many people have taken the time to share with me their experiences, knowledge and wisdom in the development of this book. They are purveyors of hope and work tirelessly in their own ways to ensure that maternity can be different for all.

Chapter 3: PERSON-CENTRED AND COMPASSIONATE LEADERSHIP

Karen Ledger is a therapist, an NHS Accredited Executive Coach, trainer and author. She is on the British Association of Counselling and Psychotherapy Executive, Coaching Division. Karen runs a busy practice, KSL Consulting, in Sheffield and London (www.karenledger. co.uk), which is a provider for the NHS Leadership Academy. Karen is the co-director of a coaching and leadership consultancy, with Jan Smith, called Between US (www.between-us.co.uk).

Jess Read is the Deputy Chief Midwifery Officer for NHS England and has been a midwife for over 30 years. Jess is a Florence Nightingale Leadership Scholar and has a strong interest in the development of a new generation of midwifery leaders.

Sheena Byrom is a freelance midwifery consultant, international speaker, author and maternity leader. She is one half of All4Maternity and *The Practising Midwife* journal. Sheena received an OBE in 2011 for services to midwifery and an Honorary Fellowship of the Royal College of Midwives in 2015.

Chapter 4: SPEAKING OUR TRUTHS

Amity Reed is a midwife, campaigner and author of *Overdue: Birth, burnout and a blueprint for a better NHS*. Originally from the US, Amity now lives in England.

Jenny Clarke is a midwifery consultant, speaker, and a huge advocate for kindness and compassion in maternity services and of skin-to-skin.

Beatrice Bennett is a third-year midwifery student at Nottingham University, a feminist, and a strong advocate for women and birthing people.

Alice Bell is a GP in London with an interest in women's health. The experience she shared was entered into the BMA's writing competition, in which she was the runner-up.

Sally Pezaro is a Fellow of the Royal College of Midwives (FRCM) and a Nursing and Midwifery Council (NMC) panellist with clinical as well as research and teaching experience. She was honoured with a first prize award from the Royal Society of Medicine in 'Leading and inspiring excellence in maternity care' and was also runner-up for the *British Journal of Midwifery*'s Midwife of the Year in 2019.

Hannah Horne is the Head of Midwifery and Gynaecology at an NHS Trust. She is also a Florence Nightingale Leadership Scholar and is passionate about providing compassionate leadership.

Ruth-Anna is an obstetrician at an NHS Trust. She fiercely believes in learning when care doesn't go as expected, and is passionate about human factors in maternity.

Nicole Rajan-Brown is a student midwife, hypnobirthing teacher and co-editor of *The Student Midwife Journal*. Nicole is fascinated by the way language works, and this important intersection with the birth experience. She is passionate about changing the culture around the language used in birth.

Chapter 7: DARE TO DREAM

Rebecca Lawton is a Professor of Psychology of Healthcare at the University of Leeds, with key interests in patient safety and lifestyle behaviour change. Rebecca is director of the Yorkshire and Humber Patient Safety Translational Research Centre and is a founder member of the Yorkshire Quality and Safety Research Group.

Tomasina Stacey is a midwife, researcher and Reader of Midwifery Practice at the University of Huddersfield. Her research interests focus on improving perinatal outcomes, in particular on the reduction of stillbirth, and quality improvement in maternity services as a whole.

Michelle Hemmington is the co-founder of the Campaign for Safer Births (CfSB) which was established, along with Nicky Lyon, in 2013. Following major errors in her care during term labour, doctors were unable to resuscitate Michelle's son Louie, and he was later registered stillborn. Their campaign has worked for over seven years to increase awareness of avoidable harm in maternity, to campaign for independent investigations with parent involvement, for coroner jurisdiction for stillbirth and for improvements in safety in maternity services.

Leila Benyounes is a barrister who specialises in clinical negligence and inquests who has represented families involved in cases where care hasn't gone as expected. Leila works for Parklane Plowden Chambers.

Benash Nazmeen is a specialist cultural liaison midwife, working towards addressing health inequalities as highlighted by MBRRACE within maternity services. She has co-designed and runs Cultural Competency and Safety Workshops for maternity healthcare professionals, while working closely with diverse communities. As a director of Sheffield Maternity Cooperative she is working to provide alternative spaces for advocacy, support and safe spaces for black and brown communities. She co-founded the Association of South Asian Midwives (ASAM), which aims to increase awareness of South Asian communities and their concerns with maternity healthcare professionals. They are also working closely to highlight and support the South Asian workforce and working with the communities to tackle taboo subjects like loss, mental health and infertility.

Billie Hunter is the RCM Professor of Midwifery. She is the director of a WHO Collaborating Centre for Midwifery Development within the WHO European Region, which focuses on strengthening midwifery throughout Europe. Billie was made a Fellow of the Royal College of Midwives in 2016 and in 2018 she was awarded a CBE in the Queen's Birthday Honours, in recognition of her services to midwifery and midwifery education in the UK and in Europe. Billie is an Honorary Professor of Midwifery in the School of Nursing, Midwifery and Physiotherapy, University of Nottingham, and an

Adjunct Professor, Faculty of Health, University of Technology Sydney (UTS), Australia. She undertakes and oversees research projects at Cardiff University.

Lucie Warren is a qualified midwife and academic at Cardiff University. She holds two posts within the School of Healthcare Sciences as a research associate working under the Maternal, Child and Family Health Research Theme, and in the Midwifery education team as a lecturer.

Sally Pezaro is a Fellow of the Royal College of Midwives (FRCM) and a Nursing and Midwifery Council (NMC) panellist with clinical as well as research and teaching experience. She was honoured with a first prize award from the Royal Society of Medicine in 'Leading and inspiring excellence in maternity care' and was also runner-up for the *British Journal of Midwifery*'s Midwife of the Year in 2019.

Jenny Patterson is a midwife and academic at Edinburgh Napier University. Jenny has a particular interest in women's traumatic birth experiences. She has been part of an international group of midwives, midwifery researchers and lecturers that has explored midwives' needs with regard to stress and trauma through workshops and surveys across the UK and Ireland. Following completion of trauma management training in 2014, Jenny has led workshops for both women and midwives.

ACKNOWLEDGEMENTS

The inspiration for *Nurturing Maternity Staff* comes from the countless individuals who have shared their experiences with me over the years, and their hope that one day the organisation they have whole heartedly committed themselves to will be better.

Many people have contributed their wisdom, experiences, and research in the making of this book, and for that I am truly grateful. Where I have used a first name, this is possibly altered to preserve anonymity. The courage, honesty, and dignity with which many staff have shared their experiences with me has been truly humbling, and inspiring.

To the amazing team I get to work with at Make Birth Better: Nikki, Emma, Sakina, Becca, Evelien, Trudi and Nat, thank you for your commitment and determination to do everything to achieve our goal to make birth better for all. Thanks also to our followers, parents and professionals, who have taught me so much about birth trauma, its ripple effect, and how the maternity system can be better.

I was so pleased when Karen Ledger, who wrote the chapter 'Person-centred and Compassionate Leadership' agreed to contribute to this book and share her wisdom. Over the years of our working together, I have learned a great deal from her, particularly about the importance of 'staying in the relationship'. I am grateful for her support and friendship.

Thank you to my wonderful husband, who champions anything I ever set out to do. His unrelenting patience in my endless dialogues about the content of this book, and skills in editing the manuscript, have been enormously helpful. For my wonderful children, I hope I make you proud, and my twin, who is one of my biggest cheerleaders. Lastly, but by no means least, to my parents; where it all began. They taught me the language of kindness, and what it means to live a life of value.

REFERENCES

INTRODUCTION: MATERNITY STAFF MATTER

1. The Royal College of Midwives, State of Maternity Services Report (2018) [Online], Available: www.rcm.org.uk/publications [Accessed 06/06/20]
2. The Royal College of Midwives, Evidence to the NHS Pay Review Body (2017), [Online], Available: www.rcm.org.uk/media/1911/rcm-evidence-nhs-pay-review-2017.pdf [Accessed 06/06/20]
3. Hunter, B., Fenwick, J., Sidebotham, M., and Henley, J. (2019). Midwives in the United Kingdom: Levels of burnout, depression, anxiety, and stress and associated predictors. *Midwifery* 79.
4. Hunter, B., Henley, J., Fenwick, J. et al. (2018). Work, Health and Emotional Lives of Midwives in the United Kingdom: The UK WHELM study. School of Healthcare Sciences, Cardiff University.
5. Fenwick, J., Hammond, A., Raymond, J., Smith, R., Gray, J., Fourer, M., Homer, C., Symon, A. (2012) Surviving, not thriving, a qualitative study of newly qualified midwives' experience of their transition to practice. *Journal of Clinical Nursing*, Volume 21.
6. Department of Health. (2012). Compassion in Practice. Nursing, midwifery and care staff: our vision and strategy. Available: www.england.nhs.uk/wp-content/uploads/ 2012/12/compassion-in-practice.pdf. Accessed 08/06/20.
7. Slade, P., Balling, K., Sheen, K., Goodfellow, L., Rymer, J., Spiby, H., Weeks, A. (2020). Work-related post-traumatic stress symptoms in obstetricians and gynaecologists: findings from INDIGO a mixed-methods study with a cross-sectional survey and in-depth interviews. *BJOG: An International Journal of Obstetrics & Gynaecology*.
8. Montgomery, A., Georganta, K., Doulougeri, K., Panagopoulou, E. (2015). Burnout: Why Interventions Fail and What Can We Do Differently. In Karanika-Murray, M. & Biron, C. (eds). *Derailed Organisational Interventions for Stress and Wellbeing*.

Chapter 1: MENTAL WELLBEING IN MATERNITY

1. Leiter, M.P., & Maslach, C. (1988). The impact of interpersonal environment on burnout and organizational commitment. *Journal of Organizational Behavior*, 9(4), 297–308.
2. Hämmig, O. (2018). Explaining burnout and the intention to leave the profession among health professionals - A cross-sectional study in a hospital setting in Switzerland. BMCC Health Services.
3. Hall, L.H., Johnson, J., Watt, I., Tsipa, A., & O'Connor, D.B. (2016). Healthcare staff wellbeing, burnout, and patient safety: A systematic review. PLoS One, 11(7), e0159015.
4. Cramer, E., & Hunter, B. (2019). Relationships between working conditions and emotional wellbeing in midwives. *Women and Birth*, 32(6), 521–532.
5. Wallbank, S., & Robertson, N. (2013). Predictors of staff distress

in response to professionally experienced miscarriage, stillbirth and neonatal loss: A questionnaire survey. *International Journal of Nursing Studies*, 50(8), 1090–1097.

6. Beck, C.T., Logiudice, J., & Gable, R.K. (2015). A mixed-methods study of secondary traumatic stress in certified nurse-midwives: Shaken belief in the birth process. *Journal of Midwifery & Women's Health*, 60(1), 16–23.

7. Hunter, 2019

8. Bourne, T., Shah, H., Falconieri, N., et al. Burnout, wellbeing and defensive medical practice among obstetricians and gynaecologists in the UK: a cross-sectional survey study. *BMJ Open* 2019;9:e030968.

9. Giménez-Espert, M.C. & Prado-Gascó, V.J. (2018). The role of empathy and emotional intelligence in nurses' communication attitudes using regression models and fuzzy-set qualitative comparative analysis models. *Journal of Clinical Nursing*, 27(13–14), 2661–2672.

10. De la Fuente-Solana, E.I., Suleiman-Martos, N., Velando-Soriano, A., Cañadas-De la Fuente, G.R., Herrera-Cabrerizo, B. and Albendín-García, L. (2020), Predictors of burnout of health professionals in the departments of maternity and gynaecology, and its association with personality factors: A multicentre study. *Journal of Clinical Nursing.*

11. Smith, J. (2020). When Two Worlds Collide: Values & Morality. *The Psychologist.*

12. Liamiani, G., Borghi, L., Argentaro, P. (2017). When healthcare professionals cannot do the right thing: A systematic review of moral distress and its correlates. *Journal of Health Psychology*, 22(1), 55-67.

13. Baptie, G., Baddeley, A., Smith, J. (2020). The Impact of COVID on Maternity Staff. *Make Birth Better.* London.

14. Rosenbaum, L. Facing Covid-19 in Italy – ethics, logistics, and therapeutics on the epidemic's front line. *New England Journal of Medicine*, 382;20, 1873-1875.

15. Litz, B.T., Stein, N., Delaney, E. et al. (2009). Moral injury and moral repair in war veterans: a preliminary model and intervention strategy. *Clinical Psychology Review*, 29, 695–706.

16. Williamson, V., Stevelink, S.A.M., Greenberg, N. (2018). Occupational moral injury and mental health: systematic review and meta-analysis. *British Journal of Psychiatry*, 212, 339–346.

17. Barnes, H.A., Hurley, R.A., Taber, K.H. (2019). Moral Injury and PTSD: Often Co-Occurring Yet Mechanistically Different. *The Journal of Neuropsychiatry and Clinical Neurosciences*, 31(2), A4-103.

18. Hunter, B., Fenwick, J., Sidebotham, M., and Henley, J. (2019). Midwives in the United Kingdom: Levels of burnout, depression, anxiety, and stress and associated predictors. *Midwifery* 79.

19. Harvie, K., Sidebotham, M., Fenwick, J., 2019. Australian midwives' intentions to leave the profession and the reasons why. *Women*

Birth.
20. Figley, C.R. Compassion fatigue: Toward a new understanding of the costs of caring. In: Stamm, B.H., ed. *Secondary Traumatic Stress: Self Care Issues for Clinicians, Researchers, and Educators.* Lutherville, MD: Sidran Press; 1995:3-28.
21. Gentry, J.E., Baranowsky, A.B., Dunning, K. ARP: The Accelerated Recovery Program for compassion fatigue. In C.R. Figley (Ed.), *Treating compassion fatigue*, Brunner-Rutledge, New York (2002), pp.123-137.

Chapter 2: WORKING IN A TRAUMATISED SYSTEM

1. Youngson, Robin (2012). *Time to Care: How to Love Your Patients and Your Job.* Rebelheart Publishers. New Zealand
2. Friedman, M.J. *Post-Traumatic Stress Disorder* (Compact Clinicals, Kansas City, 2001).
3. Dahlen, H.G. & Caplice, S. (2014). What do Midwives Fear? *Women and Birth,* 27, 266-70. *NHSS* Resolution. Annual report and accounts 2018/2019. 2019. https://assets.publishing.service.gov.uk/government/uploads/system/uploads/attachment_data/file/824345/NHS_Resolution_Annual_Report_and_accounts_print.pdf
4. Magro, M. Five years of cerebral palsy claims: a thematic review of NHS Resolution data. 2017. https://resolution.nhs.uk/wp-content/uploads/2017/09/Five-years-of-cerebral-palsy-claims_A-thematic-review-of-NHS-Resolution-data.pdf
5. Goldstone, A.R., Callaghan, C.J., Mackay, J., Charman, S., Nashef, S. (2004). Should surgeons take a break after an intraoperative death? Attitude survey and outcome evaluation. *BMJ*, 328:379
6. Lewis, G., & Drife, J. (2004). Confidential Enquiry into Maternal and Child Health: Improving care for mothers, babies, and children. Why Mothers Die 2000–2002. The Sixth Report of the Confidential Enquiries into Maternal Deaths in the United Kingdom. *Royal College of Obstetricians and Gynaecologists.* London.
7. Macdonald, M., Gosakan, R., Cooper, A.E., Fothergill, D.J. Dealing with a serious incident requiring investigation in obstetrics and gynaecology: a training perspective. *The Obstetrician & Gynaecologist* 2014;16:109–14.
8. Pezaro, S., Pearce, G. & Bailey, E. 2018, Childbearing women's experiences of midwives' workplace distress: Patient and Public Involvement *British Journal of Midwifery,* 26 (*10*), pp.659-669.
9. Litorp, H., Mgaya, A., Mbekenga, C.K., Kidanto, H.L., Johnsdotter, S., Essen, B. (2015). Fear, blame and transparency: Obstetric caregivers' rationales for high caesarean section rates in a low-resource setting. *Social Science & Medicine, (143),* 232-240.
10. Birchard, K. (1999). Defence union suggest new approach to handling litigation costs in Ireland. *Lancet,* 354:1710.
11. Edmondson, A.C. (1999). Psychological Safety and Learning Behavior in Work Teams. *Administrative Science Quarterly,* 44,

350-383.

12. Brown, B. (2012). *Daring Greatly. How the Courage to be Vulnerable Transforms the Way we Live, Love, Parent, and Lead*. Penguin Life. London.
13. West, M.S., and Chowla, R. (2017). Compassionate leadership for compassionate healthcare. In Gilbert, P. (Ed). *Compassion: concepts, research, and applications*. London. Routledge, 237-257.
14. Make Birth Better Model. http://makebirthbetter.org

Chapter 3: PERSON-CENTRED AND COMPASSIONATE LEADERSHIP

1. Rogers, C. (1961). On Becoming a Person: A Therapist's View of Psychotherapy, page 284. London: Constable.
2. Atkins PWB, Parker SK (2012). 'Understanding individual compassion in organisations: the role of appraisals and psychological flexibility'. Academy of Management Review, vol 37, no 4, pp 524–46.
3. West, MA & Chowla, R 2017, Compassionate leadership for compassionate health care. in P Gilbert (ed.), Compassion: Concepts, Research and Applications. Routledge, London, pp. 237-257.

Chapter 4: SPEAKING OUR TRUTHS

1. Camden Coalition of Healthcare Providers in New Jersey
2. MerseyCare Just Culture
3. Kivimaki, M., et al. (2001). Sickness absence in hospital physicians: a 2-year follow-up study on determinants. *Occupational and Environmental Medicine*, 58(6), 361-366.
4. Jill Maben et al., 2012. Exploring the relationship between patients' experience of care and the influence of staff motivation, affect, and wellbeing. [pdf] Available at: www. nets.nihr.ac.uk/__data/assets/pdf_file/0007/85093/ES-08-1819-213.pdf
5. The Point of Care (2019). Impact Report: How the Point of Care Foundation's programmes support healthcare staff and patients.
6. Lown, B.A., Manning, C.F. The Schwartz center rounds: evaluation of an interdisciplinary approach to enhancing patient-centered communication, teamwork, and provider support. *Academic Medicine* 2010;85:1073–81.
7. Goodrich, J. Supporting hospital staff to provide compassionate care: do Schwartz Center Rounds work in English hospitals? *J R Soc Med* 2012;105:117–22.
8. Taylor, C., Xyrichis, A., Leamy, M.C., et al. Can Schwartz Center Rounds support healthcare staff with emotional challenges at work, and how do they compare with other interventions aimed at providing similar support? A systematic review and scoping reviews. *BMJ Open* 2018;8:e024254. doi:10.1136/ BMJ open-2018-024254.
9. Pearson, Q.M. (2004). Getting the most out of clinical supervision: Strategies for mental health counselling students. *Journal of Mental Health Counseling*, 26(4), 361–373.

10. Mackin, P., Sinclair, M. (2003) Labour ward midwives' perceptions of stress. *Journal of Advanced Nursing* 27(5): 986-91.
11. Kenardy, J.A. The current status of psychological debriefing. *BMJ* 2000;321:1032
12. Rimmer, A. What should I eat on my night shift? *BMJ* 2019; 365 doi: https://doi.org/10.1136/bmj.l2143 (Published 16 May 2019)
13. Chatfield, C., Rimmer, A. Give us a break. *BMJ* 2019;364:l481.
14. Available from: http://www.mentalhealth.org. UK/publications. Mental Health Foundation— Be Mindful Report, United Kingdom, 2010.
15. Gu, J., Strauss, C., Bond, R., & Cavanagh, K. (2016). How do mindfulness-based cognitive therapy and mindfulness-based stress reduction improve mental health and wellbeing? A systematic review and meta-analysis of mediation studies: Corrigendum. *Clinical Psychology Review, 49,* 119. https://doi.org/10.1016/j.cpr.2016.09.011
16. Babette Rothchild (2006). *Help for the Helper: the psychophysiology of compassion fatigue and vicarious trauma.* W.W. Norton & Company. New York.

Chapter 5: THE TIDE OF CHANGE

1. MerseyCare Just Culture. Available at https://www.merseycare.nhs.uk/about-us/restorative-just-and-learning-culture
2. NHS England (2020). *Just and learning culture central to improving care.* NHS Merseycare Foundation Trust.
3. Kivimaki, M., et al. (2001). Sickness absence in hospital physicans: 2 year follow up study on determinants. *Occupational and Environmental Medicine*, 58(6), 361-366.
4. Jill Maben et al, 2012. Exploring the relationship between patients' experience of care and the influence of staff motivation, affect and wellbeing. [pdf] Available at: www. nets.nihr.ac.uk/__data/assets/pdf_file/0007/85093/ES-08-1819-213.pdf
5. The Point of Care (2019). Impact Report: How the Point of Care Foundation's programmes support healthcare staff and patients.
6. Lown BA, Manning CF. The schwartz center rounds: evaluation of an interdisciplinary approach to enhancing patient-centered communication, teamwork, and provider support. *Acad Med* 2010;85:1073–81.
7. Goodrich J. Supporting hospital staff to provide compassionate care: do Schwartz Center Rounds work in English hospitals? J R Soc Med 2012;105:117–22.
8. Taylor C, Xyrichis A, Leamy MC, et al. Can Schwartz Center Rounds support healthcare staff with emotional challenges at work, and how do they compare with other interventions aimed at providing similar support? A systematic review and scoping reviews. BMJ Open 2018;8:e024254. doi:10.1136/ bmjopen-2018-024254.
9. Pearson, Q. M. (2004). Getting the most out of clinical supervision: Strategies for mental health counselling students. *Journal of Mental Health Counseling*, 26(4), 361–373.

10. Mackin P, Sinclair M. (2003) Labour ward midwives' perceptions of stress. *Journal of Advanced Nursing* 27(5): 986-91.
11. Kenardy JA. The current status of psychological debriefing. *BMJ* 2000;321:1032
12. Rimmer, A. What should I eat on my night shift? BMJ 2019; 365 doi: https://doi.org/10.1136/bmj.l2143 (Published 16 May 2019) *BMJ* 2019;365:l2143
13. Chatfield C, Rimmer A. Give us a break. *BMJ* 2019;364:l481.
14. vailable from: http://www.mentalhealth.org. uk/publications. Mental Health Foundation – Be Mindful Report, United Kingdom, 2010.
15. Gu, J., Strauss, C., Bond, R., & Cavanagh, K. (2016). "How do mindfulness-based cognitive therapy and mindfulness-based stress reduction improve mental health and wellbeing? A systematic review and meta-analysis of mediation studies": Corrigendum. *Clinical Psychology Review*, 49, 119. https://doi.org/10.1016/j.cpr.2016.09.011
16. Babette Rothchild (2006). *Help for the Helper: the psychophysiology of compassion fatigue and vicarious trauma.* W.W. Norton & Company. New York.

Chapter 6: EMBRACING DIFFERENCE

1. Edmondson, A.C., Woolley, A.W. Understanding outcomes of organizational learning interventions. In: Easterby-Smith, M., Lyles, M., (eds). *Blackwell handbook of organizational learning and knowledge management*. Malden: Blackwell Publishing; 2003.
2. Edmondson, A. (1999). Psychological safety and learning behavior in work teams. *Administrative Science Quarterly*, 44(2), 350-383.
3. Delizonna, L. (2017). High-performing teams need psychological safety. Here's how to create it. *Harvard Business Review*, 8, 1-5.
4. Riskin, A., P. Bamberger, A. Erez, T. Foulk, B. Cooper, I. Peterfreund, J. Sheps, M. Wilhelm-Kafil, Y. Riskin, K. Riskin-Guez and E. Bamberger (2019). Incivility and Patient Safety: A Longitudinal Study of Rudeness, Protocol Compliance, and Adverse Events. *The Joint Commission Journal on Quality and Patient Safety* 45(5): 358-367.
5. Royal College of Midwives, Royal College of Obstetricians and Gynaecologists. Each baby counts the 2019 progress report. htttps://tinyurl.com/u3zb912 (accessed 28 October 2020) Google Scholar.
6. Hunter, B. (2001). Emotion work in midwifery: a review of current knowledge. *Journal of Advanced Nursing* 34(4): 436-444.
7. Hunter, B., Warren, L. (2014) Midwives' experiences of workplace resilience. *Midwifery* 30 (2014) 926-934.
8. Hunter, B., Warren, L. (2015) Caring for ourselves: the key to resilience In: Downe, S., Byrom, S. *The Roar Behind the Silence: Why kindness, compassion and respect matter in maternity care.* London, Pinter & Martin pp111-115

9. Health Education England (HEE). 2018. RePAIR: Reducing Pre-registration Attrition and Improving Retention Report. London: HEE.
10. West, M., Bailey, S., Williams, E. 2020 The Courage of Compassion. Kings Fund, London.
11. Pezaro, S., Clyne, W. and Fulton, E.A. A systematic mixed-methods review of interventions, outcomes and experiences for midwives and student midwives in work-related psychological distress. *Midwifery* (2017). DOI: http://dx.doi.org/10.1016/j.midw.2017.04.003
12. Herzog, J.I. and Schmahl, C. (2018) Adverse Childhood Experiences and the Consequences on Neurobiological, Psychosocial, and Somatic Conditions Across the Lifespan. *Frontiers in Psychiatry* 9:420
13. Mental Health Taskforce NE. The Five Year Forward View for Mental Health. 2016
14. Raja, S., Hasnain, M., Hoersch, M., Gove-Yin, S., Rajagopalan, C. & Kruthoff, M. Trauma-Informed Care in Medicine: Current Knowledge and Future Research Directions. *Family and Community Health*. 2015 Jul-Sep;38(3):216-26.
15. NHS Education for Scotland. (2013). One out of Four Learning Resource. Retrieved from www.knowledge.scot.nhs.uk/maternalhealth/learning/one-out-of-four.aspx
16. Walsh, D.J. (2011). Nesting and Matrescence. In R. Bryar & M. Sinclair (Eds.), *Theory for Midwifery Practice* (2nd ed.). Basingstoke: Palgrave MacMillan.

Chapter 7: DARE TO DREAM

1. NHS Staff Survey (2020). National NHS Staff Survey Co-Ordination Centre (https://www.nhsstaffsurveyresults.com, accessed 29th May 2021).
2. Edmondson AC, Woolley AW. Understanding outcomes of organizational learning interventions. In: Easterby-Smith M, Lyles M, editors. *Blackwell handbook of organizational learning and knowledge management*. Malden: Blackwell Publishing; 2003.
3. Edmondson, A. (1999). Psychological safety and learning behavior in work teams. *Administrative science quarterly*, 44(2), 350-383.
4. Delizonna, L. (2017). High-performing teams need psychological safety. Here's how to create It. *Harvard Business Review*, 8, 1-5.
5. Riskin, A., P. Bamberger, A. Erez, T. Foulk, B. Cooper, I. Peterfreund, J. Sheps, M. Wilhelm-Kafil, Y. Riskin, K. Riskin-Guez and E. Bamberger (2019). "Incivility and Patient Safety: A Longitudinal Study of Rudeness, Protocol Compliance, and Adverse Events." *The Joint Commission Journal on Quality and Patient Safety* 45(5): 358-367.
6. Royal College of Midwives, Royal College of Obstetricians and Gynaecologists. Each baby counts, 2019 progress report. htttps://tinyurl.com/u3zb912 (accessed 28 October 2020) Google Scholar
7. Hunter, B. (2001). "Emotion work in midwifery: a review of current knowledge." *Journal of Advanced Nursing* 34(4): 436-444.

8. MBRRACE-UK (2020). Saving Lives, Improving Mothers' Care.
9. MBRRACE-UK (2019). Saving Lives, Improving Mothers' Care.
10. MBRRACE-UK (2014). Saving Lives, Improving Mothers' Care.
11. Hunter B, Warren L (2014) Midwives' experiences of workplace resilience. *Midwifery* 30 (2014) 926-934
12. Hunter B, Warren L (2015) Caring for ourselves: the key to resilience in Downe S, Byrom S *The Roar Behind the Silence: Why kindness, compassion and respect matter in maternity care.* London, Pinter & Martin pp 111-115.
13. Health Education England (HEE). 2018. RePAIR: Reducing Pre-registration Attrition and Improving Retention Report. London: HEE.
14. West M., Bailey S., Williams E. 2020 The Courage of Compassion. Kings Fund, London.
15. Pezaro, S. (2016). The midwifery workforce: A global picture of psychological distress – Article in *Midwives: Official journal of the Royal College of Midwives*, 19:33
16. Pezaro, S. (2016). Addressing psychological distress in midwives. *Nursing Times, 112*, (8), 22-23.
17. Pezaro, S., Clyne, W., Turner, A., Fulton, E. A., & Gerada, C. (2015). 'Midwives overboard! 'Inside their hearts are breaking, their makeup may be flaking but their smile still stays on. *Women and Birth* 29.3: e59-e66.
18. Pezaro, S, Clyne, W and Fulton, E.A (2017). "A systematic mixed-methods review of interventions, outcomes and experiences for midwives and student midwives in work-related psychological distress." *Midwifery.*
19. NHS Health Scotland (2019). Adverse Childhood Experiences in Context. (www.healthscotland.scot, accessed 29/01/21).
20. Mind (2020). Mental Health Facts and Statistics (www.mind.org 21/01/21).
21. Sheela, R., Memoona, H., Hoersch, M.,Gove-Yin, S., Rajagopalan, C. (2015). Trauma Informed Care in Medicine, *Family & Community Health*, 38(3), 216-226.
22. NHS Education for Scotland. (2013). One out of Four Learning Resource. Retrieved from www.knowledge.scot.nhs.uk/maternalhealth/learning/one-out-of-four.aspx
23. Walsh, D., J. (2011). Nesting and Matrescence. In R. Bryar & M. Sinclair (Eds.), *Theory for Midwifery Practice* (2nd ed.). Basingstoke: Palgrave MacMillan.

INDEX